THE RIDER'S FITNESS PROGRAM

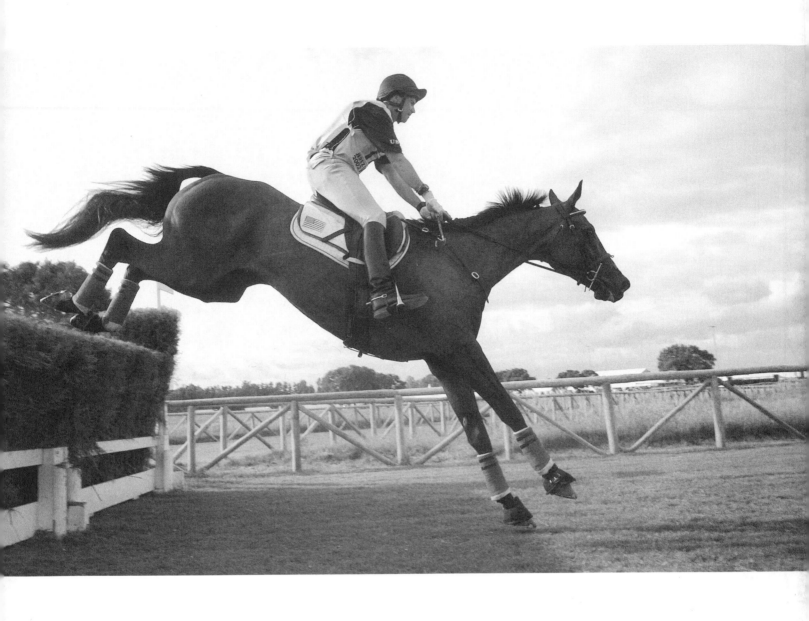

THE RIDER'S FITNESS PROGRAM

74 Exercises & 18 Workouts Specifically Designed for the Equestrian

Foreword by Anne Kursinski

DIANNA ROBIN DENNIS • JOHN J. McCULLY • PAUL M. JURIS

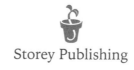

Storey Publishing

The mission of Storey Publishing is to serve our customers by publishing practical information that encourages personal independence in harmony with the environment.

Edited by Deb Burns and Siobhan Dunn
Art direction by Melanie Jolicoeur and Vicky Vaughn
Cover and text design by Melanie Jolicoeur and Vicky Vaughn
Cover photographs © Shaffer Smith Photography: front cover bottom three, back cover left; © Kit Houghton/CORBIS: front cover top; back cover right.
Excercise photographs © Shaffer Smith Photography
Additional interior photographs © Alamy Images: 64; © Kent Barker/The Image Bank/Getty: 18; © Digital Vision/Getty: 108; © Sharon P. Fibelkorn: 168; © Kit Houghton/CORBIS: viii; © Charles Mann Photography: ii, 136; © Mike Powell/The Image Bank/Getty: x; © Nicholas Russell/The Image Bank/Getty: 40; © Shaffer Smith Photography: v center.
Text production by Vicky Vaughn
Indexed by Eileen Clawson
Fitness models: Lori Matan, Tracy Jetzer, and Aimee Steele
Illustrations by James Dykeman

The information in this book is true and complete to the best of our knowledge. All recommendations are made without guarantee on the part of the authors or Storey Publishing. The authors and publisher disclaim any liability in connection with the use of this information. For additional information, please contact Storey Publishing, 210 MASS MoCA Way, North Adams, MA 01247.

Storey books are available for special premium and promotional uses and for customized editions. For further information, please call 1-800-793-9396.

Printed in the United States by Vicks Lithograph
10 9 8 7 6 5 4 3 2 1

Library of Congress Cataloging-in-Publication Data
Dennis, Dianna R.
    Rider's fitness program: 74 fitness exercises specifically designed to help you improve physical fitness, increase strength, and achieve oneness with your horse / Dianna Robin Dennis, Johnny J. McCully, and Paul M. Juris.
        p. cm.
    Includes bibliographical references and index.
    ISBN 1-58017-542-2 (pb : alk. paper)
1. Horsemanship. 2. Physical fitness. I. McCully, John J. II. Juris, Paul M. III. Title.

RC1220.H67D46 2004
613.7'1—dc22
                                        2004018551

DEDICATION

Dedicated to our horses — who love us when we are fit and, sometimes, tolerate us when we aren't.

To my father, who supported me, believed in me, made a personal investment in my future, and never gave up. Thanks, Dad.

To Lisa, Sam, and Sydney, my wonderful family and daily inspiration, whose passionate love of animals introduced me to the equestrian world.

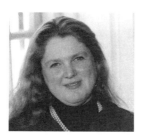

Dianna Robin Dennis

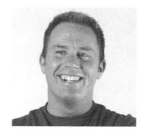

John J. McCully

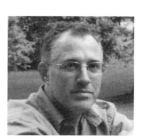

Paul M. Juris

CONTENTS

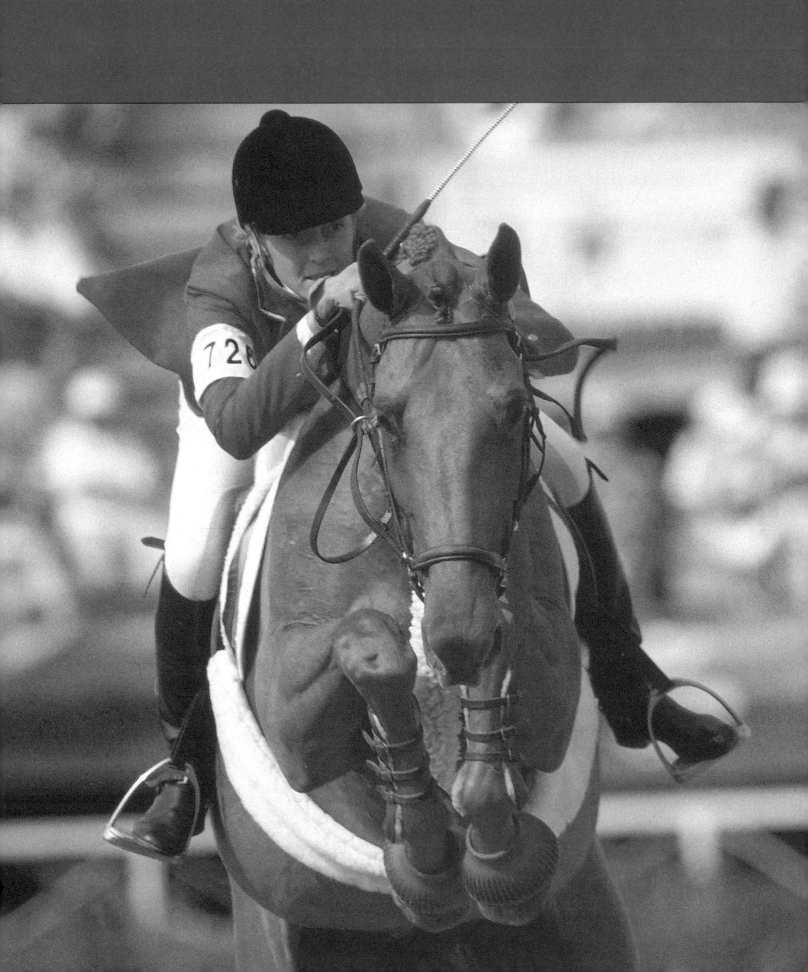

FOREWORD

Years ago I didn't believe I needed an exercise program. I thought riding and jumping horses all day was enough.

I knew my horses needed to be fit to compete at the highest levels; I knew fitness made them stronger, sounder, more supple, more balanced/lighter — more athletic overall — but I never realized this also applied to me.

After my first Olympics Games, and after being around all those "real athletes" in the other sports, I started my first workout "program". It was pretty eye opening for me, an Olympian, to be working out with the average gym-goer, but, as my business grew, I put working out on the back shelf. After all, I was an Olympian, and I had ridden umpteen horses a day every day since I started riding at age four — I didn't believe working out could make such a difference to me.

Then, injury struck, and my knee specialist told me I didn't need an operation, I needed a proper exercise program. I'd been using the same muscles for riding all my life and my body needed to be more "balanced". While I understood what he meant, I didn't really see it, until I watched a friend training for the New York Marathon, with Johnny McCully. This was my first exposure to "sport-specific exercise".

Johnny and Paul Juris spent hours with me — videotaping my students and me, analyzing our performances, and developing this program. I use it; my students use it.

It makes a difference — not only for those of us at the highest levels, but especially for those who are only weekend or occasional riders — from amateurs who work at a desk during the week and compete on weekends to those who want to go for that once a year week-long ride on the beaches of Majorca!

We riders and our equine partners need to be strong, supple, and generally fit to prevent injury and to maximize our performance. If one member of this partnership is tired, she won't be able to communicate with the other member! That could lead to something as simple as a time fault or rail down to something as serious as a crash.

The goal for all riders is to achieve that ultimate feeling of "oneness" with our horses.

This fitness program makes that goal more attainable for all of us!

— *Anne Kursinski*

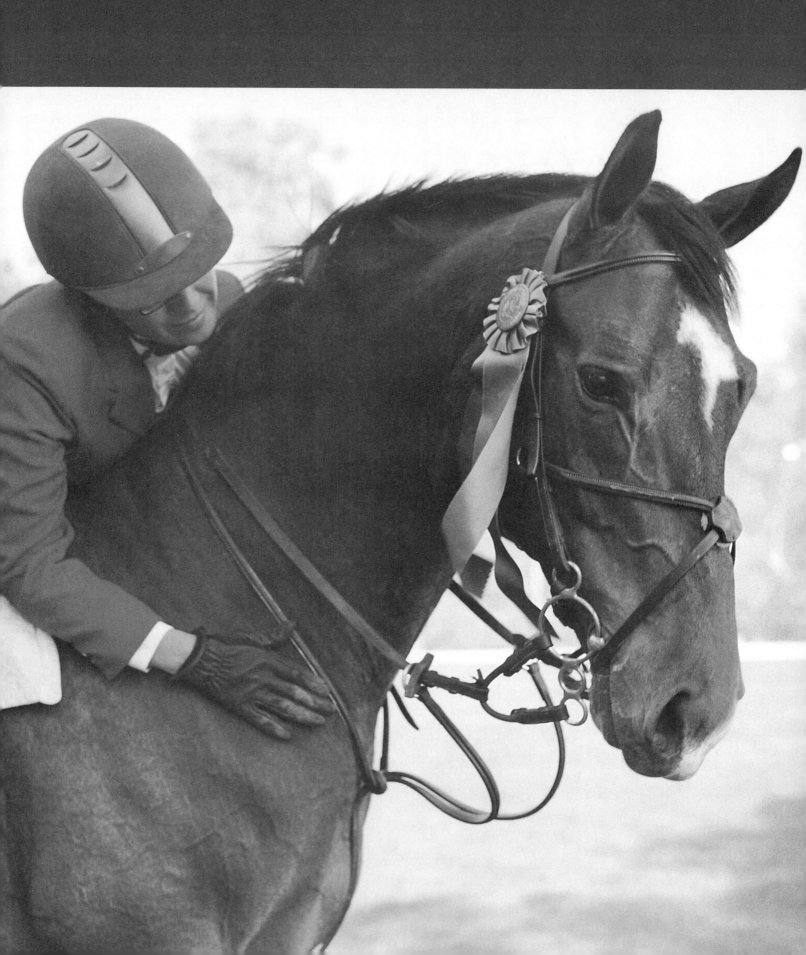

THE PROGRAM

What kind of rider are you? What is your discipline? Are you a beginner, an expert, or somewhere in the vast middle? Regardless of your level, fitness will help you, your performance, and your communication with your horse.

The goal of every rider is "oneness" with the horse. Oneness may mean something different for each of us who rides, but most would agree it is the feeling of coordination, balance, and communication that comes when you and your horse are on the same wavelength and going in the same direction.

An unfit rider — unfit physically, mentally, or emotionally — cannot achieve oneness. You may strive for it, but to get there, all the pieces of the puzzle must be in place. To ride the best you can, your muscles, ligaments, coordination, balance, and brain must all be working as well as possible.

For beginners and low-level riders, a proper fitness regimen, created specifically for riding, will alleviate many of the aches and pains associated with getting started, as well as prevent injury. For the rider coming back to the sport after a long hiatus, this program will help recall those all-important body memories and lessen the time needed to get back where you once were. For the expert, this will hone your skills and help prevent injury, especially as you get older.

The exercises and routines that constitute our program were developed with riders at a variety of levels and disciplines through observation and video analysis. It is appropriate for:

- beginners — regardless of discipline
- those who jump — hunter, jumper, steeplechase
- those who ride on the flat — pleasure, dressage, reining
- competitive event riders, who do all three disciplines
- polo players
- endurance riders
- those who ride for fun or infrequently

Although each of these disciplines may have a slightly different emphasis, they all demand the same basic fitness skill set.

CRITICAL ELEMENTS OF EQUESTRIAN FITNESS

There are five basic elements to equestrian fitness:

- Balance
- Flexibility
- Strength
- Mental/physical independence
- Aerobic (cardiovascular)

Balance

How stable are you as a rider? How long does it take for your muscles to tire? How well can you maintain your center of gravity (COG) when your horse is moving? Can you hold your "half-seat" or "galloping position" for lengths of time at any gait? How is your sitting trot? Can you adapt your position to instantly respond to any problem? Can you adjust your position to save your horse when his balance becomes precarious, as he sometimes adjusts for you?

Riding and aligning yourself with your horse's COG is what creates the "oneness" we all strive for as riders. We are using the technical term *core stability* to describe how stable you are on your horse, even though this term has multiple meanings in the sport fitness world. Of course, finding your core stability is far easier practiced on the ground than mounted!

Flexibility

Functional flexibility, or the flexibility that is required to perform the functions of a task, is often overlooked. It is critical to your longevity as a rider. The simple act of mounting is an excellent way to test your functional flexibility.

Mounting and dismounting demand a specific set of muscles to make the acts quick, easy, and balanced (not disturbing the horse). The flexibility required to get your leg over your horse without excessively rounding out your lumbar spine and tilting your pelvis is often neglected, and if not maintained can lead to back, hip, and other joint problems.

Strength

Strength is, of course, the most easily recognized, but often the most misunderstood, aspect of fitness. Many people associate strength with how much weight they can lift or how large their muscles appear. Unfortunately, neither of those characteristics translates into improved performance on a horse. *Strength* can best be defined as the ability to apply force, and in the equestrian environment, that means applying force on a moving animal to which one's attachments are the stirrups, saddle, and reins. Along with aerobic conditioning, strength training is most often part of regular, non-sport-specific fitness programs. In the horse world, strength is essential and must be combined with flexibility and balance.

Mental/Physical Independence

We don't think of riding as similar to walking, scratching our head, chatting on the cell phone, and chewing gum simultaneously, but it is — and much more.

Riders both act and process information simultaneously; the legs, arms, shoulders, back, seat, head, and so forth are usually doing different things. Asymmetric movement refers to unequal or different movement on either side of the body. Not only do riders have to be able to act asymmetrically, but they also must be able to do a number of different physical and mental tasks at one time. This is called multitasking.

If you must think about using your arms and legs in separate movements, it will detract from your overall performance and

The primary issue for rider fitness and balance is that your posture is dynamic — you and your horse are in constant motion, which, in turn, places more demand on your natural and achieved balance. For our purposes, we call this your *core stability*.

There are five mechanisms that make up core stability — **center of gravity; stability; power; symmetric posture**; and **asymmetric movement, stability** and **strength.** The muscles that make up your body's core are found in your back and abdomen — strengthening these muscles contributes to overall fitness and stability.

Center of gravity

Your center of gravity will impact your balance, how you ride, and how you need to compensate in your riding. For example, a long-torso, short-legged rider, with a high center of gravity needs to be much stronger in the back and must be aware of the impact her upper-body motion will have on balance and the horse's movement, especially when jumping.

Stability

Your hips, knees, and ankles — also known as plantar stabilizers and hip abductors (shock absorbers) — are primary areas where there can never be too much flexibility, strength, and control.

Your pelvic absorption must be efficient and effective, coordinating the hips, pelvis, and lumbar spine. A flexible, strong lower back is essential. The focus is not only short-term stability, but also prevention of long-term orthopedic problems.

Power

In addition to absorbing, you need to transmit energy produced by your horse. Transmitting describes how you use the energy generated by your horse (especially in jumping when your horse meets the ground). It critically affects horse/rider efficiency, or "oneness."

Symmetric posture

Your body needs to be even and square. Just as straightness and forwardness in a horse are building blocks, the even and balanced development of your body, as your horse's partner, is also critical. Most of us, just like our horses, favor one side or another and part of proper fitness is evening up our two sides.

Asymmetric movement, stability, and strength

Most rider/horse communication is asymmetric, from bending your horse around your inside leg, with the outside leg behind the girth, to slightly moving one hip/seat bone to cue a flying change. All are imperceptible, necessary, and asymmetric.

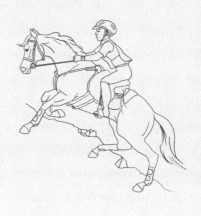

"oneness" with the horse. The ability to automatically and independently manipulate each hand and arm is a trainable skill.

Any rider, especially one jumping cross-country at speed, has to gauge and process a myriad of external information at once and, by processing it, use it to perform his or her best. For example, galloping toward a series of fences, you notice a deep muck hole caused by the riders before you. Can you avoid this without making too much or too obvious a change? Can you immediately understand how it will impact your horse's jump and make the appropriate changes to your riding? Can you do it so automatically and quickly that you don't even know you are doing it? That is our goal.

Closed and Open Skills

Part of refining our processing skills is understanding the "open" and "closed" skills required for riding.

A closed skill is highly predictable; the conditions do not change. Therefore, the training required for a closed skill involves perfecting the predictable task. There are some elements of riding that are closed. For example, your jumps don't move, and you can dictate their height. Your dressage test or reining pattern is set, and the movements required have a specific "correct" execution.

Most of what we do in riding is considered an open skill: highly unpredictable and rapidly changing. To perform well, you must be able to recognize, understand, and react to the rapidly changing nature of your task. Of course, communicating with your horse is an open skill, as the horse is an entity in and of itself. You can never overestimate the unpredictability of the horse!

Rapid multitasking exercises enhance your effectiveness as a rider; however, these exercises should be done after you achieve ease and consistency in the simpler components of this program. This stage of "automaticity" training helps your ability to be "in the zone" and is an advanced tactic used in the third cycle of training.

Remember, it is critical for you to concentrate when doing your exercises. They lose their effectiveness when you perform them by rote, as nothing in riding is done by rote.

Aerobic (Cardiovascular) Fitness

Aerobic or cardiovascular fitness is important to your ability to sustain an activity. Can you complete a long jumper course with an immediate jump-off without losing your breath? Can you gallop your horse for 5 miles — with or without jumps? Can you walk your cross-country course once, much less four times, without getting winded?

Although performing our routines without rest does improve your aerobic fitness to some degree, we encourage you to add walking, jogging, running, biking, or swimming to your fitness program. For land-based activities, it is especially important to incorporate hillwork when possible.

Other Fitness Issues

We horse people supplement our horses' feed with both preventive and supportive minerals and nutrients. However, we ourselves

WHAT IS YOUR CENTER OF GRAVITY?

We all talk about center of gravity, but do we really understand what it is and how it affects us as riders?

Your center of gravity is the balance point in your body. The major segments of your body — trunk, arms, legs, and head — all have different masses. The average of these masses is located just behind your navel when you're standing upright. That is your center of gravity, the location of the average mass of your body.

Think of a seesaw: When the two ends of the seesaw are balanced, the fulcrum — center — is the center of gravity. What happens when a heavier person sits on one end? The balance is lost, and the center of gravity moves toward the heavier side, pulling down that side and pushing up the opposite side. If the heavier person moves toward the center, the balance is regained, and the center of gravity returns to the seesaw center, or fulcrum.

Your center of gravity as a rider is determined by your size, shape, and fitness. A person with heavy bones and muscle will have different issues from someone who is skin and bones. A horse's center of gravity is dependent on his gait and frame or degree of collection. A fully collected dressage horse will have a center of gravity that is higher and more vertical than that of a fully galloping racehorse.

For you, as the rider, this means that your center of gravity is dynamic; it changes with your horse's gait, balance, and speed. Your own center of gravity needs to match and influence that of your horse. The closer you are to always being centered over your horse, the closer you are to achieving "oneness" and staying with your horse when there is a sudden movement, problem, or "out-of-balance" situation.

tend to live on diet soda and hotdogs!

Part of any fitness program is proper nutrition. For riders, especially, care must be taken to ensure development and repair of bone, muscle, ligament, and tendon fiber and structure. This means a balanced diet supplemented with vitamins and minerals that work to maintain and protect our bodies.

We strongly suggest that you find a doctor who is well versed in athletes' needs and practices and is familiar with both the benefits and the pitfalls of supplements. Given that broken bones are almost a norm rather than

an unusual occurrence in riding, we especially stress getting your bone density checked regularly — regardless of your age — and make sure your calcium, potassium, and magnesium levels are being maintained.

Supplements will help your brain and your body when you are horse showing, particularly when you are on the run and not able to eat. However, there is no substitute for good nutrition and a balanced diet. As an athlete, you need to drink plenty of water — especially when competing in the heat. Remember, if you *feel* thirsty, you are already dehydrated!

TOOLS, CLOTHING, AND EQUIPMENT

Wear comfortable clothes with shoes that properly support your feet. As you improve, and the exercises get easier, you can add the challenge of doing them in your helmet (especially important for your balance) and breeches and boots (for your flexibility or lack thereof, depending on the fit!).

We have tried to suggest at-home alternatives to all the exercises designed for gym machines. Many of these alternative setups can already be found in your home or barn, and we have included some sources on our Web site www.ridinghighfitness.com

Basic Home Equipment:

- **Mat.** It is always helpful to get a good padded mat; however, a towel or carpeting will suffice.
- **Bands.** These come in two styles: straight with two ends, and round (like an oversized rubber band). They also come in an assortment of strengths, so you can change (increase) the tension.
- **Physioball.** This large blow-up ball is used to add the challenge of instability to a seated exercise.
- **Medicine ball.** This heavy round ball, rather like a cannonball, comes in various sizes and weights.
- **Weight bar.** This approximately 3-foot-long, heavy bar comes in a variety of weights.
- **Small blocks.** A child's building blocks, cut 4 × 4's, or even riding Blox will do.
- **Dumbbells.** A variety of weights from 5 to 20 pounds is recommended.
- **Bench/chair.** Just make sure it is heavy and stable enough to be safe!
- **Incline board.** A table or board, raised on one end, is used for increasing the difficulty of seated or lying-down exercises.
- **Tilt board.** This board on a roller demands that you have good balance to remain steady. Very useful in the multitasking exercises.
- **Step stools.** One with and one without wheels will be useful.
- **Ankle & wrist weights.** To wrap these around your ankles or wrists, secure with Velcro. They can be used for some routines or when walking/running to increase the difficulty.
- **Three-foot-long, half-round foam rollers.** These are for balance and stability exercises; they can also be used to stretch your back!

SAFETY

What if something hurts? Analyze the pain. Is it an "ouch" pain, meaning you have stressed or torn something? Or is it the feeling of your muscles saying, "Oh, this is too hard?" If it is the "ouch" kind, stop immediately and seek professional advice. If it is the difficulty of exertion, disregard the adage "No pain, no gain"; retreat a little from what you are doing, then slowly build back to that point. Seeking the advice of a professional trainer is always helpful.

Basic gym equipment, in addition to the home equipment listed at left, includes:

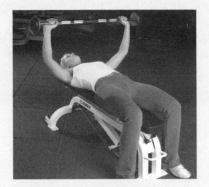

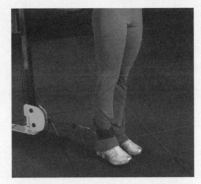

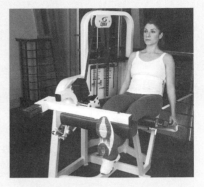

Utility benches. These are readily available in most gyms. They are either fixed flat or adjustable to several incline positions. Find a comfortable and stable bench for your exercises. Make sure it's wide enough, but not so wide as to restrict motion.

Pulley systems, or cable columns, also widely used in gyms today. They may be fixed pulleys, in which the pulleys are anchored at the top and bottom of the machine, or adjustable, in which the pulley may be moved.

A leg extension machine. This is a standard device for strengthening the knee extensor muscles in the front of the thigh. Find one that allows you to sit comfortably with your knee joint aligned with the rotating axis of the machine.

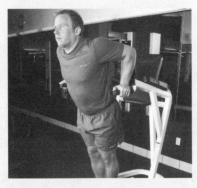

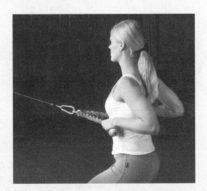

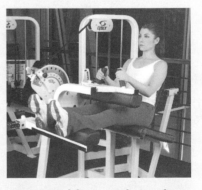

Parallel dip bars, in many shapes and sizes. Some are freestanding, and others come as part of large multi-gym systems with weight assistance. Use one that fits and supports your frame or provides assistance as you gain strength through these movements.

Pulley system with twin rope handle. This is the same as those described above, except that it is always adjustable. The height of the pulley should be adjusted so that it is level with the shoulder. The rope handles allow for unrestricted motion of the arms.

A seated leg curl machine. This is the counterpart of the leg extension. The knees should again be aligned with the rotational axis of the device and the support pad should be positioned low on the calf, without touching the Achilles tendon.

THE ROUTINES

The heart of our program lies in the series of routines matching skill-based exercises with up-to-date athletic training methods. We have spent hundreds of hours working with riders and watching videos in order to create a dynamic exercise program. We've analyzed the fitness needs of riders at a variety of levels and disciplines, both casual and competitive, and our routines are custom-created to meet the needs of any rider, regardless of ability. Our unique, six-week sequence of routines creates a complete, riding-specific workout program that benefits the horseback rider by developing both fitness and skill levels.

Why So Many Routines?

The Rider's Fitness Program differs from other programs because of the specific sequence of eighteen different routines of five to seven exercises each, performed over a six-week period. Why not do the same routine for six weeks, as many programs suggest? We have found, both through our work in the fitness field and through scientific research, that adaptation to a routine occurs very quickly. In other words, your body gets used to a repeated routine, and after a period of time — sometimes as short as two weeks — very little is gained. This is due to the body's ability to memorize and adapt to, or stop learning from, repetitive movement.

The most effective means of physical fitness training is to continually require the body to do new things, thus forcing it to adapt and develop new skills. Our program of varied routines does just that, leading to more extensive and long-lasting gains in motor skills.

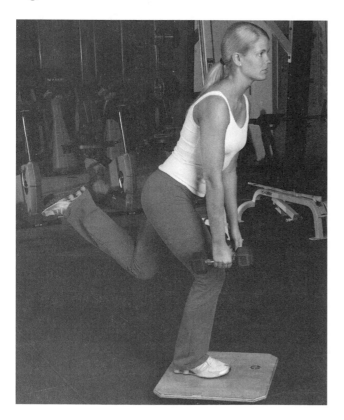 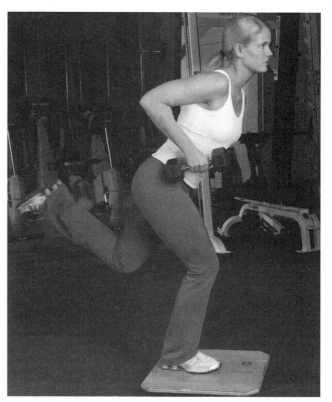

Unlike body building programs, we are not interested in how much weight you use when you do the exercises. The best place to start is with a weight that, at the end of ten repetitions, makes you aware that you have done it. The last two reps should feel difficult but you should be able to complete the range of motion. If you can't quite complete the final rep or two of a set, then you are doing too many. If you feel a lower weight is too easy, before automatically increasing the weight, consider slowing down the exercise and focusing; try performing it with your full concentration. It may be that you are doing the exercise too quickly and not paying enough attention to form.

As you progress and begin the second six weeks of the program, you can use heavier weights for increased resistance or use lighter weights and do the exercises a little more quickly. Your muscles, joints, ligaments, and tendons will respond rapidly to small increases in the intensity and duration of the exercises or reps performed.

The exercises that make up the routines are based on research that tells us multi-jointed, large-muscle exercises use the most energy. Thus, the routines start with large-muscle exercises and move to exercises that focus on the smaller muscles, with balance work that includes joint movement and equal distribution of exercises on both sides of your body. Start with two sets of seven to ten repetitions each — you can, depending on how you feel, increase that over time to as many as three sets of fifteen.

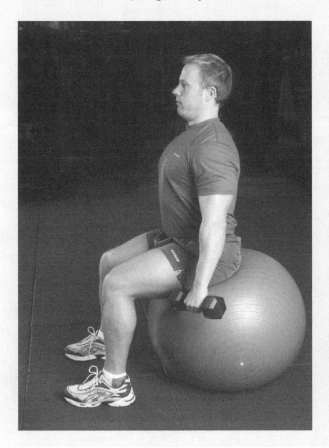

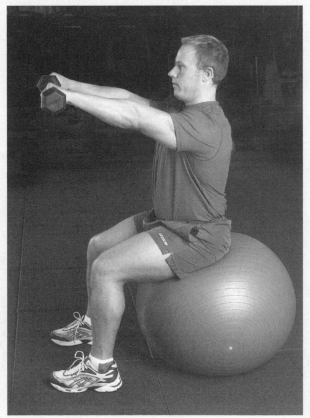

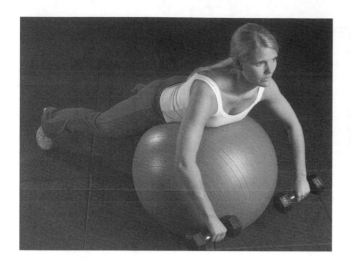
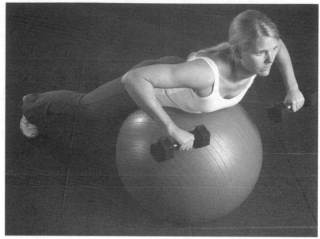

Building Skills

Riding is a set of skills, and this program was developed specifically to relate to those skills. The program is not aesthetic; the skills developed here will not make you look like a body builder. Nor are these skills measured in isolation; this isn't about winning a one-time event. The benefits of this program are realized through enhanced performance while riding. When you repeat a single routine, you reinforce only motor skills that are highly regular, fixed, predictable, and stable. This is useful in activities like bowling and darts, where the environment is fixed and stable, but riding, of course, is entirely different! The dynamic, variable, and unstable skills required by horseback riding are promoted and enhanced by routines that are equally dynamic, variable, and, sometimes, even unbalanced. This is the basis for the program.

The fact that no two days' routines are identical promotes your mental awareness and concentration. Furthermore, these routines emphasize skills that are used by all riders, no matter their fitness level or type of riding. Whether you are developing new skills or enhancing them through training, our program will make you a more effective rider.

Looking at the charts on the following pages, you will see six blocks each containing three routines. Each block represents one week of training, and each routine, one day in the week. You can do the workouts on any three days of the week, according to your own schedule, taking off one or two days between sessions. We have included a detachable chart of the routines at the back of the book. Use it to record your workouts, sets and repetitions, and weights.

A THREE-PHASE PROGRAM

The six weeks are divided into two-week segments. The first two weeks are the "Intro" phase, when you start conditioning your body. You'll accustom your body to performing different routines and exercises and at the same time work on the building blocks that will allow you to perform the increasingly challenging tasks that follow.

The second phase of our program introduces more difficult exercises, some of which concentrate on two actions simultaneously.

These are focused skill-building exercises that lead to the final two weeks' challenges, which increase the variables as well as the difficulty of each routine's exercises.

Continuing Fitness

When you have finished the sixth week, you can start over: Increase, decrease, or vary your weights and/or your velocity using the weights, and increase your repetitions and sets. As you become more familiar with the program and how to use it over a six-week period, you can create your own organization of routines to match your changing needs. If you have found some exercises easy and some more difficult, you may need to change an exercise, keeping in mind that the variation or replacement exercise should be from the same section as the original.

Remember, this isn't about memorizing the exercises and performing them by rote; it is about concentrating and teaching your body how to react so that it can respond quickly and automatically to riding challenges.

Planning a Successful Workout

Organize yourself ahead of time — plan your week to work out Monday, Wednesday, and Friday or Tuesday, Thursday, and Saturday. The important thing is to be consistent and to take days off in between. Here are some suggestions:

- Try to keep to the same schedule for the entire six-week period.
- Find the weight and the number of reps and sets that is right for you and stick to it for the length of the program. If you feel that the exercises are too easy, focus on your performance before automatically increasing the weight or reps.
- Have all your equipment and gear ready so you can work through the routines without stopping.
- Warm up before and stretch after each workout.

STRETCHING

Stretching after any physical workout benefits your mind and body in many different ways:

- By improving circulation and increasing blood flow to the muscles and tendons.
- By increasing your heart rate, blood pressure, and temperature — literally warming you up!
- Rotation stretches increase your range of motion as well as the speed of muscular contractions. Stretching prepares the neuromuscular pathways for more intense activity.
- Slow stretching loosens tense muscles and tendons and helps reduce the risk of injury as well as stiffness and soreness.
- Proper stretching improves the flexibility of the lumbar and pelvic areas, thus reducing the risk of pain in the lower back.
- Stretching will help to focus your mind, regulate your breathing, and balance your body.
- Stretched muscles and tendons are relaxed, improving the flexibility you gain through the workout.

WEEK ONE

Routine One

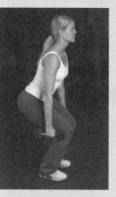

Exercise	Chapter
12 | Squat	Lower Body
24 | Hip abduction	Lower Body
31 | Seated heel raise at horse width	Lower Body
66 | Reverse-grip pull-down	Upper Body
62 | Close-grip bench press	Upper Body
74 | Upright row	Upper Body
54 | Trunk extension	Posture

Routine Two

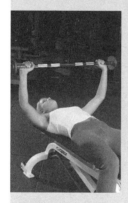

Exercise	Chapter
16 | Leg press at horse width	Lower Body
28 | Leg extension	Lower Body
29 | Seated leg curl	Lower Body
61 | Bench press	Upper Body
73 | Incline dumbbell row	Upper Body
74 | Upright row	Upper Body
34 | Incline board reverse curl	Pelvic Tilt

Routine Three

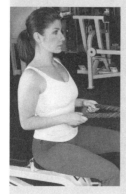

Exercise	Chapter
17 | Step up	Lower Body
25 | Hip adduction	Lower Body
69 | Standing Row, Half-Seat Position	Upper Body
68 | Straight-arm pull-down	Upper Body
74 | Upright row	Upper Body

Add Stool Scoot warm-ups to this routine for a complete workout, page 27.

Routine Four

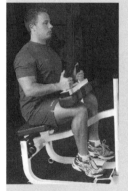

Exercise	Chapter
16	Leg press at horse width	Lower Body
24	Hip abduction	Lower Body
31	Seated heel raise at horse width	Lower Body
70	Seated row, prone grip	Upper Body
73	Incline dumbbell row	Upper Body
74	Upright row	Upper Body

Add Crunches to this routine for a complete workout, page 27.

Routine Five

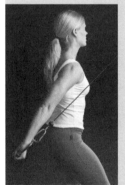

Exercise	Chapter
12	Squat	Lower Body
25	Hip adduction	Lower Body
29	Seated leg curl	Lower Body
68	Straight-arm pull-down	Upper Body
63	Close-grip bench press, feet up	Upper Body
74	Upright row	Upper Body
55	Trunk extension with rotation	Posture

Routine Six

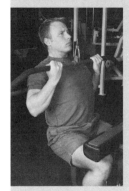

Exercise	Chapter
17	Step up	Lower Body
28	Leg extension	Lower Body
29	Seated leg curl	Lower Body
66	Reverse-grip pull-down	Upper Body
61	Bench press	Upper Body
74	Upright row	Upper Body
34	Incline board reverse curl	Pelvic Tilt

WEEK TWO

PHASE 2 BUILDING SKILLS

Routine Seven

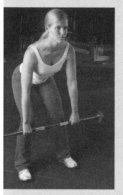

Exercise	Chapter
18 | Anterio-lateral step up	Lower Body
24 | Hip abduction	Lower Body
27 | Bent-knee dead lift	Lower Body
71 | Bent-over row	Upper Body
2 | Incline dumbbell press with feet up	Balance
33 | Hanging knee raise	Pelvic Tilt
41 | Pelvic clock	Pelvic Tilt

Routine Eight

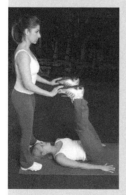

Exercise	Chapter
13 | Squat at horse width	Lower Body
16 | Leg press at horse width	Lower Body
31 | Seated heel raise at horse width	Lower Body
63 | Close-grip bench press, feet up	Upper Body
48 | Seated row on physioball	Posture
39 | Alternate leg lowering on an incline board	Pelvic Tilt
40 | Dynamic pelvic control	Pelvic Tilt

Routine Nine

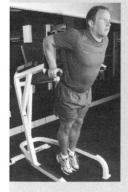

Exercise	Chapter
19 | Lateral step up	Lower Body
24 | Hip abduction	Lower Body
27 | Bent-knee dead lift	Lower Body
67 | Dips	Upper Body
47 | Seated dumbbell front raise on physioball	Posture
43 | Seated physioball back and forth	Pelvic Tilt
41 | Pelvic clock	Pelvic Tilt

Routine Ten

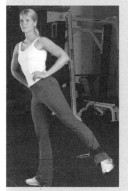

Exercise	Chapter
13 | Squat at horse width	Lower Body
11 | Cable pull-through with one-leg stance	Balance
32 | Half-seat raise	Lower Body
48 | Seated row on physioball	Posture
46 | Shoulder rotation with physioball	Posture
43 | Seated physioball back and forth	Pelvic Tilt
60 | Self-mobilization with physioball and foam roller	Posture

Routine Eleven

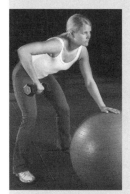

Exercise	Chapter
19 | Lateral step up	Lower Body
10 | Standing hip extension	Balance
26 | Straight-knee dead lift	Lower Body
47 | Seated dumbbell front raise on physioball	Posture
72 | Bent-over transverse row	Upper Body
42 | Seated physioball hula	Pelvic Tilt
45 | Trunk extension with rotation on physioball	Pelvic Tilt

Routine Twelve

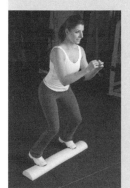

Exercise	Chapter
13 | Squat at horse width	Lower Body
22 | Forward leg swing	Lower Body
32 | Half-seat raise	Lower Body
68 | Straight-arm pull down	Upper Body
47 | Seated dumbbell front raise on physioball	Posture
45 | Trunk extension with rotation on physioball	Pelvic Tilt
42 | Seated physioball hula	Pelvic Tilt

WEEK FOUR

WEEK FIVE

Routine Thirteen

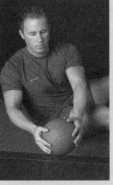

Exercise	Chapter
7 ǀ Horse-width squat on half-round	Balance
8 ǀ Unilateral squat	Balance
30 ǀ Standing heel raise at horse width with angulation	Lower Body
46 ǀ Shoulder rotation with physioball	Posture
50 ǀ Russian twist with medicine ball	Posture
54 ǀ Trunk Extension	Posture

Routine Fourteen

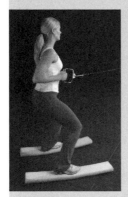

Exercise	Chapter
14 ǀ Squat at horse width with lateral shift	Lower Body
3 ǀ Cable row in half-seat on a half-round	Balance
56 ǀ Medicine ball swing	Posture
58 ǀ Quadruped trunk extension	Posture
37 ǀ Trunk curl with rotation on a physioball	Pelvic Tilt
1 ǀ Reciprocal dumbbell press	Balance

Routine Fifteen

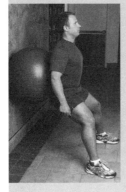

Exercise	Chapter
15 ǀ Timed wall squat with physioball	Lower Body
20 ǀ Lunge	Lower Body
30 ǀ Standing heel raise at horse width with angulation	Lower Body
72 ǀ Bent-over transverse row	Upper Body
38 ǀ Trunk curl with alternate knee raise on physioball	Pelvic Tilt
51 ǀ Side plank	Posture

Routine Sixteen

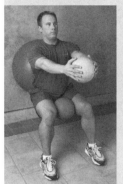

Exercise	Chapter
49	Timed wall squat with trunk rotation	Lower Body
23	Standing hip extension with external rotation	Lower Body
64	Medicine ball push-up	Upper Body
6	Upright row on one leg	Balance
52	Side plank on DynaDisc	Posture

Routine Seventeen

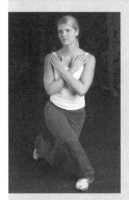

Exercise	Chapter
14	Squat at horse width with lateral shift	Lower Body
21	Crossover lunge	Lower Body
4	Half-seat cable row with two tilt boards	Balance
56	Medicine ball swing	Posture
59	Prone trunk extension on physioball with shoulder extension	Posture
36	Counter rotation	Pelvic Tilt

Routine Eighteen

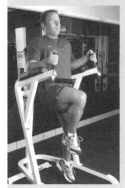

Exercise	Chapter
57	Combo squat with low-to-high pull	Posture
9	Circle hop	Balance
5	Single-leg bent-over dumbbell row on tilt board	Balance
65	Walkover push-up	Upper Body
44	Physioball scale	Pelvic Tilt
35	Reciprocal hanging knee raise	Pelvic Tilt

WEEK SIX

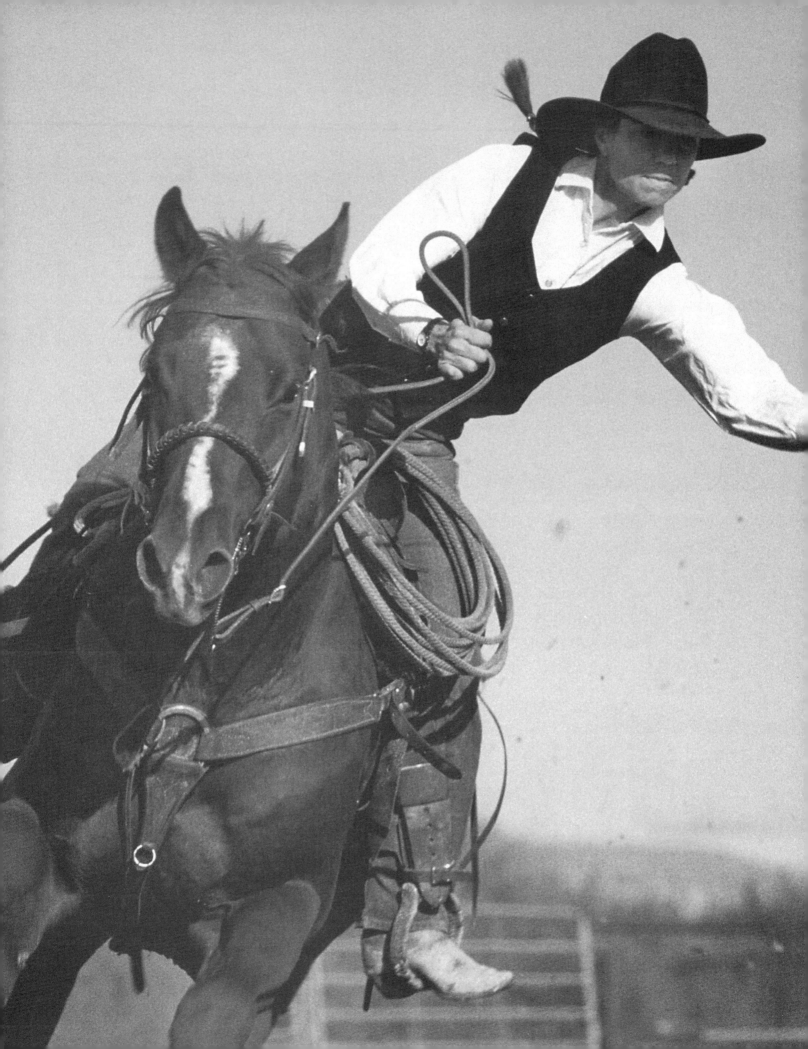

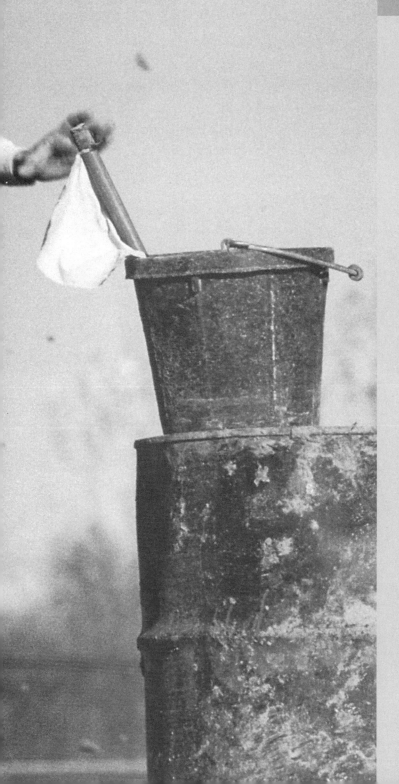

Chapter 1

WARMING UP AND STRETCHING

Warming up and stretching are important components of your exercise and riding routines. Having your muscles warmed, relaxed, and ready to work helps to prevent injury.

Some of these stretches have mounted versions that can be done on your horse when you are feeling tight and stressed or as a warm-up for a class or lesson. They can also help you relax and feel more secure in the saddle. As you get more comfortable with them, you can do them on a longed horse. You'll find them on a detachable card at the back of the book.

Maintaining mental relaxation while riding your horse is easier if you are physically relaxed and your muscles are warmed up. It also helps prevent further tightening of your body, especially when you haven't ridden in a while.

Remember to breathe when doing your stretches — on or off your horse!

Lower-Leg Stretch

How do I do this?

1. Stand barefoot 20 to 36 inches from a wall. Reaching forward, place your hands on the wall.

2. Keep your back straight and bend only at your elbows and ankles; keep both heels on the floor.

3. Continue to lean forward until you feel a slight stretch in your calf muscles. Hold for 15 to 30 seconds. Release.

4. Repeat the stretch three times.

THE ACHILLES TENDON AND GASTROCNEMIUS

The Achilles tendon extends from your heel, meeting the gastrocnemius muscle at the back of your upper calf. These tend to be very tight and can inhibit your ability to put your weight on your heels and allow your ankle to act as a shock absorber.

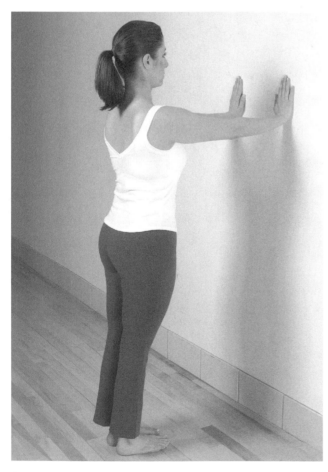

Starting position.

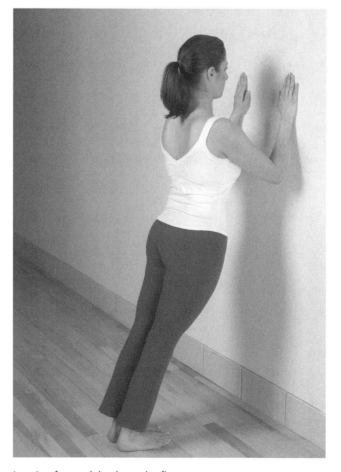

Leaning forward, heels on the floor.

Standing Quad Stretch

How do I do this?

1. Stand facing the wall, with your left hand placed on the wall for balance.

2. Bend the right leg and grasp your ankle from behind with the right hand.

3. Gently bring your heel toward the buttocks. As you slowly pull your heel toward your buttocks, move your thigh until it is directly under your pelvis, in line with your supporting leg, knee pointing to the ground. Take care not to hyperextend your lower back.

4. Hold the leg for 15 to 30 seconds, then release.

5. Repeat the stretch three times on each leg.

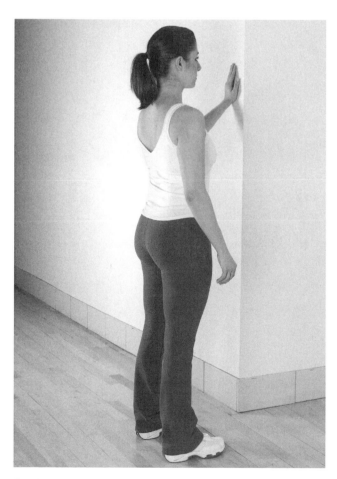

Starting position.

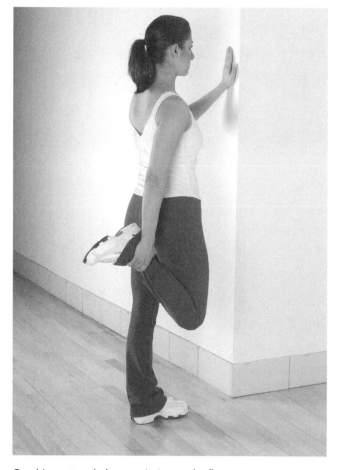

Quadricep stretch, knee pointing to the floor.

Hamstring Stretch 1

How do I do this?

1. Locate a doorway with walls on either side of the door frame, or a corner with a free wall on each side. Lying on your back, position yourself so that the outer thigh of one leg extends through the doorway or alongside the base of the wall running parallel to your leg. Your hip joint should touch the corner of the wall or door frame.

2. Raise the opposite leg, straighten the knee, and bring it across the extended leg, keeping both hips on the floor.

3. Progress the stretch by moving the leg farther across the wall toward the floor. Keep your foot pointed away from the wall as you straighten your leg. Be careful not to bounce the knee. Hold steady for 15 to 30 seconds.

4. Repeat three times with each leg.

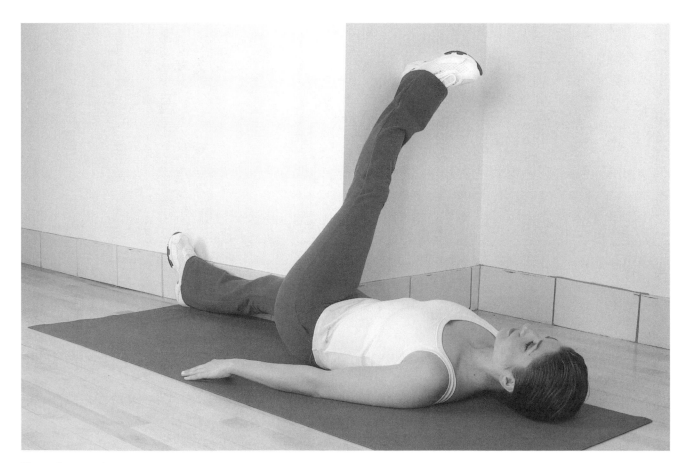

Hamstring stretch.

Hamstring Stretch 2

How do I do this?

1. Lying on your back, position yourself so that the inner thigh of one leg extends through the doorway or alongside the base of the wall running parallel to your leg. The inner thigh of the extended leg touches the door frame or the base of the parallel wall.

2. Place the opposite heel against the perpendicular wall. Slide your heel up the wall, straightening your knee and trying to bring your thigh in contact with the wall. Keep your extended leg and both hips on the ground.

3. When the leg is straight and you feel the stretch, hold for 15 to 30 seconds.

4. Repeat three times with each leg. The closer you move your hips and buttocks toward the perpendicular wall, the more intense the stretch.

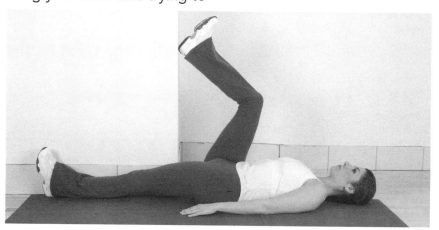

Starting position.

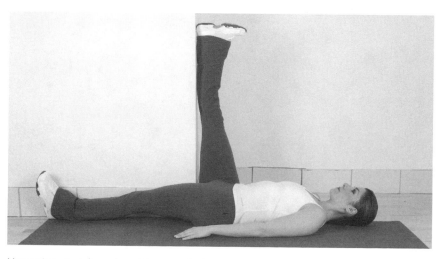

Hamstring stretch — do not bounce the knee.

Hips and Buttocks Stretch 1

How do I do this?

1. Lie flat on your back with your knees bent and feet flat on the floor.

2. Cross the right ankle onto the left knee.

3. Reach through your legs; grab behind the left knee.

4. Slowly bring the left knee toward your chest. Feel the stretch in the right buttock and hip. Hold for 15 to 30 seconds.

5. Repeat stretch three times on each side, alternating sides.

STRETCHES FOR HIPS, BUTTOCKS, AND LOWER BACK

Riding, and even simply working around horses, puts intense pressure on your hips, buttocks, and lower back. Stretching these areas before working out or riding will help you relax when mounted, as well as helping to prevent injury.

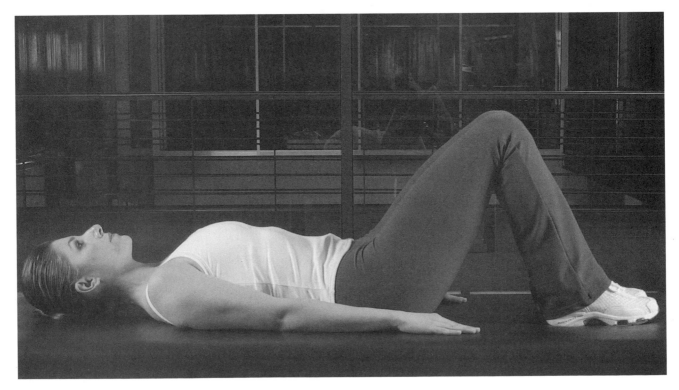

Starting position.

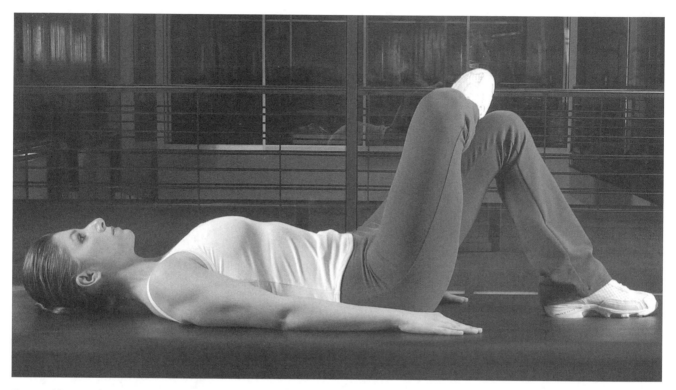

Cross ankle over the opposite knee.

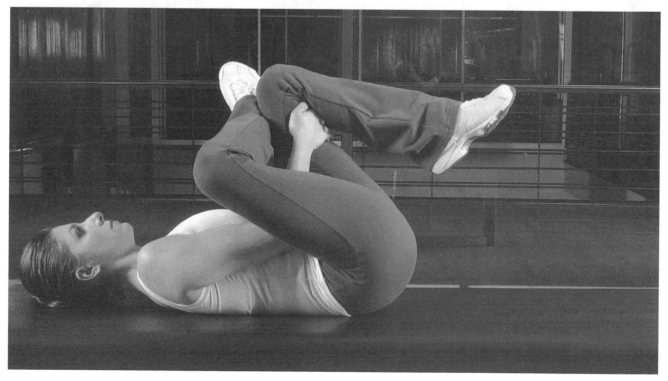

Hold the knee toward the chest.

Hips and Buttocks Stretch 2

How do I do this?

1. Lie on your right side with both legs extended.

2. Keeping your left leg straight, slowly raise it 12 to 18 inches. Be sure to keep your body still, without rolling backward or forward.

3. Slowly lower your leg to resting position.

4. Repeat the stretch in sets of seven on each side. To deepen the stretch, use a 2-pound ankle weight on the lifting leg. Build up to three sets of fifteen.

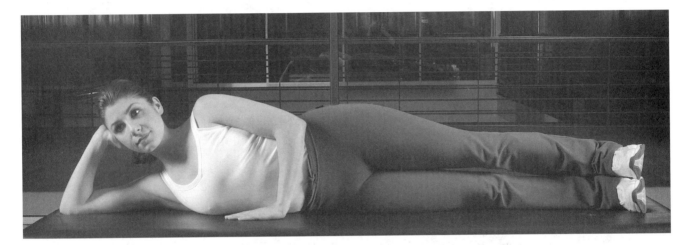

Starting position.

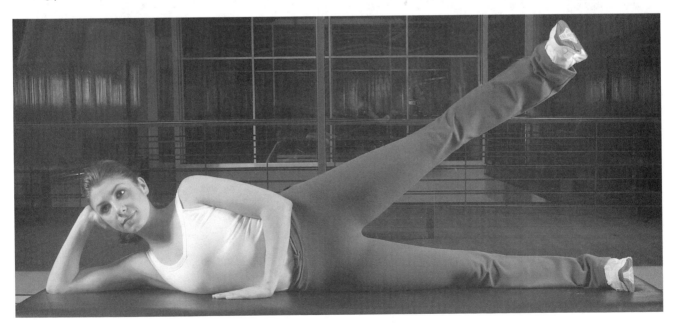

Leg raise — the feet are flexed and both legs are straight.

STOOL SCOOTS

Stool scoots develop strength around your knee joint as well as postural control. This supports your posting, your half-seat, and your galloping position, as well as helping to prevent knee-stress injuries related to riding. They are easily added to your workout and can be done in the gym, barn, or home.

- You need a stool with wheels — a kitchen stool that locks under weight will not work; a piano stool is perfect, and an office chair will do.
- Sit tall and extend both your legs. Place your feet on the floor approximately 2 feet in front of you.
- Place your hands on top of your thighs to support your body weight.
- Pull yourself and the stool/chair toward your feet. Repeat this action until you have moved about 15 feet.
- Turn around and do the same thing back. If you are in an office, use this technique to move yourself around.
- Lean forward very slightly to enhance muscular contraction.

ABDOMINAL CRUNCHES

Crunches help develop trunk and pelvic stability, which comes in handy when your horse spooks or surges forward. Add them to your regular routine. Tips for the perfect crunch:

- Lie on your back, with your legs bent and feet flat on the floor. Cross your arms over your chest and slowly raise your upper body until your shoulders are a few inches off the floor. Hold, then slowly release without totally relaxing your abdominal muscles. Repeat ten to fifteen times for three sets.
- Exhale as you rise; inhale on release.
- Add difficulty with a rotation. Curl your upper body to the right or left, alternating left elbow toward right knee, right elbow toward left knee.
- For a bicycle maneuver, place hands on either side of your head and elevate knees. Begin a slow pedaling movement with your legs. Bring the right elbow toward the left knee, then the left elbow to the right knee as you pedal. Keep the movement slow and controlled.
- Regardless of how you vary the crunch, keep your head and neck relaxed and in a natural position. Your stomach and pelvis muscles should be doing all the work, not your neck. Think about the thrust you feel when your horse suddenly moves to one side or lands over a fence.
- Opening your mouth while doing this exercise can help keep your head and neck relaxed — say "Whoa!"

Hip Extension, Prone

How do I do this?

1. Lie on your stomach with your legs straight and your chin resting on your arms.

2. Slowly lift your right leg from the floor as high as possible.

3. Slowly return the leg to the floor, pause, and relax.

4. Perform three sets of seven, alternating the legs.

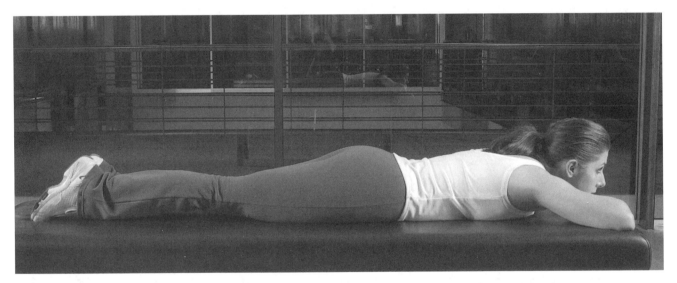

Starting position.

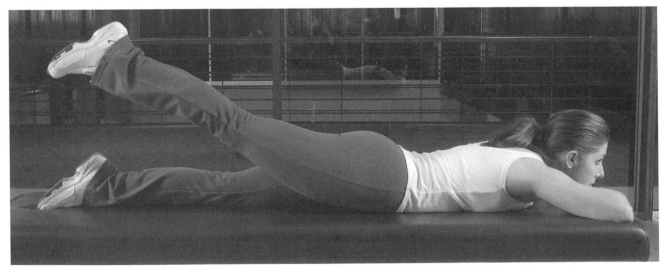

Raise leg slowly, extending from hip.

Lower-Back Stretch

How do I do this?

1. Lying on your back, bend your knees and place both feet flat on the floor.

2. Lift the knees. Wrap your arms around your bent legs and pull them toward your chest, flattening your lower back to the floor. Hold for 15 to 30 seconds.

3. Repeat three times.

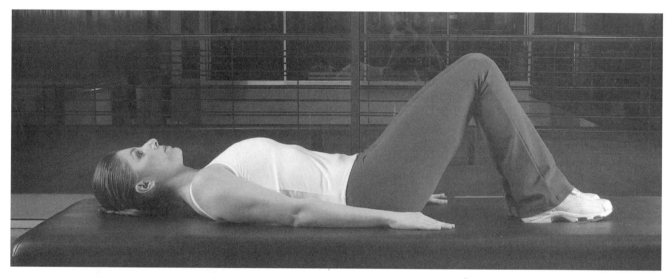

Starting position.

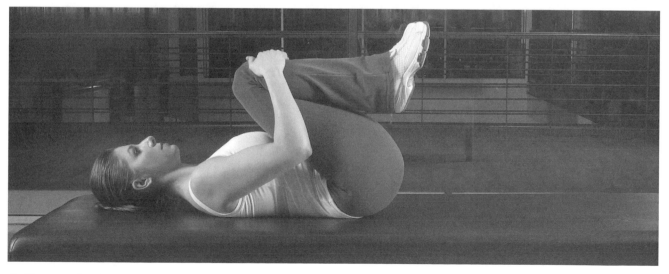

Curl knees to the chest.

Posture Stretch

How do I do this?

1. Stand in a doorway with your elbow at shoulder height. Place your palm against the doorjamb or outer wall.

2. Lean forward gently while bringing your shoulder blades together. Hold for 15 to 30 seconds.

3. Release, then return to starting position.

4. Repeat three times on each side.

SHOULDER, UPPER-BACK, AND ARM STRETCHES

Riding posture tends to be overlooked, particularly because it is difficult to maintain. Stretching the muscles of your shoulders, neck, and upper arms helps you to reduce the tension that inevitably develops in those areas when riding, especially competitively.

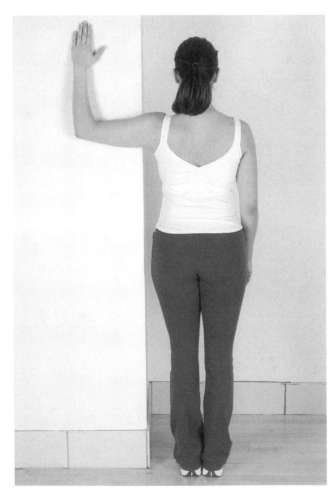

Starting position.

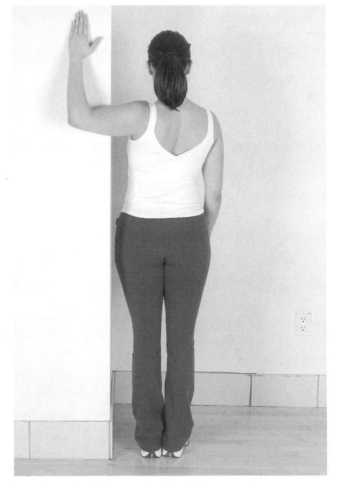

Lean forward to bring the shoulder blades together.

Neck and Shoulder Stretch

How do I do this?

1. Lie on your stomach on a bench or bed, with one arm hanging down to the side and your thumb pointing out.

2. Slowly raise the arm as high as you can, making sure the motion is centered at the shoulder blade.

3. Bring the arm back to starting position.

4. Perform seven to ten times, alternating the arms.

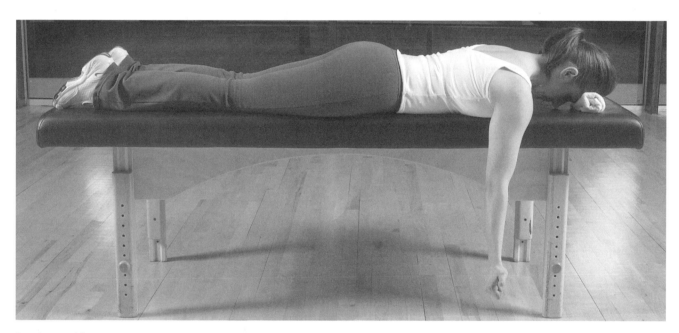

Starting position.

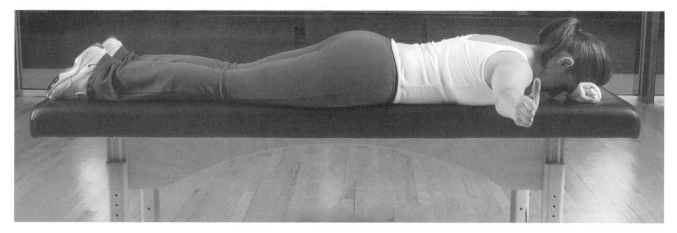

Arm raise — arm is in line with or slightly higher than the shoulders.

Shoulder Shrugs, Prone

How do I do this?

1. Lie on your stomach on a bed or bench, with one arm hanging off the side.

2. Grasp a 2.5- to 5-pound weight in your hand.

3. Slowly raise the weight, lifting from the shoulder blade and bending the elbow toward the ceiling. Keep the arm close to your side.

4. Return to starting position.

5. Perform seven to ten times with each arm.

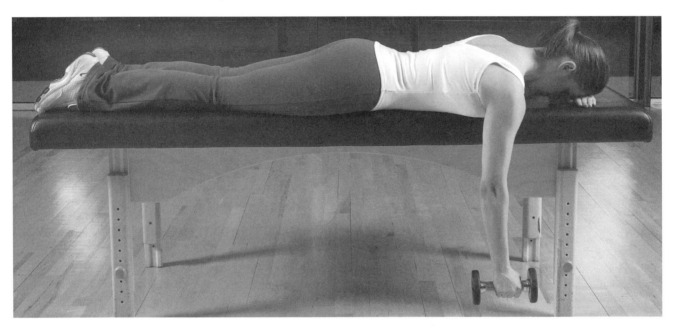

Starting position.

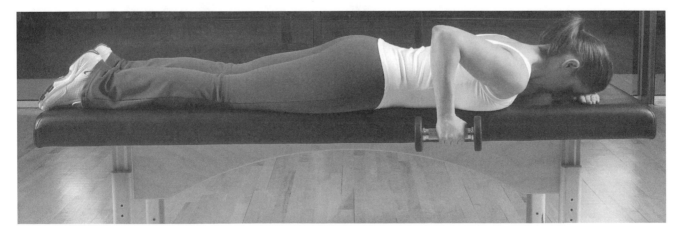

Bend at the elbow. Arm stays close to the side as you lift.

External Rotation with Elastic Resistance

How do I do this?

1. Attach an elastic exercise band to the handle of a closed door.

2. Stand with your left side next to the door.

3. Place a small pillow or rolled towel between your right arm and rib cage.

4. Grasp the elastic in your right hand and, with your arm bent at the elbow, pull the band out to the side by rotating from the shoulder.

5. Try to keep your elbow at your side and the towel in place, moving only your lower arm.

6. Perform seven to ten times with each arm.

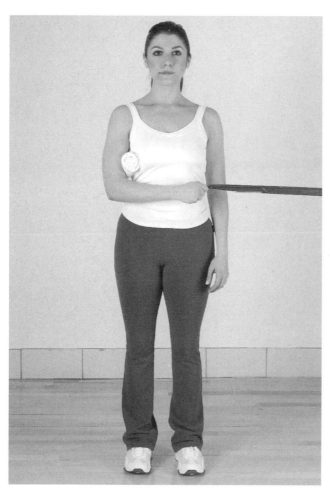

Starting position.

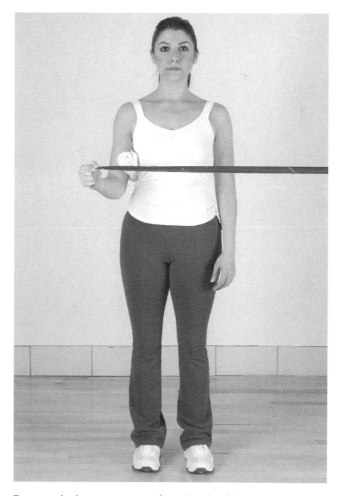

To move the bent arm, rotate from the shoulder.

Internal Rotation with Elastic Resistance

How do I do this?

1. Attach an elastic exercise band to the handle of a closed door.

2. Stand with your right side next to the closed door.

3. Place a small pillow or rolled towel between your right upper arm and rib cage.

4. Grasp the elastic in your right hand and, with your thumb pointing up and your right elbow at your side, pull the elastic across your body by rotating from the shoulder.

5. Slowly return to starting position.

6. Perform seven to ten times with each arm.

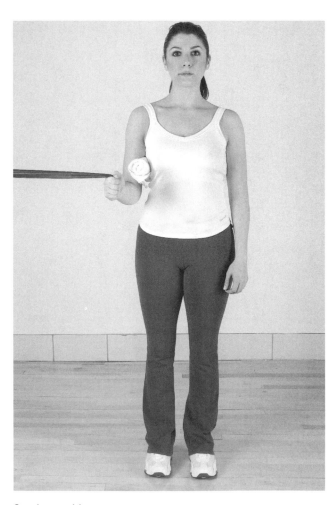

Starting position.

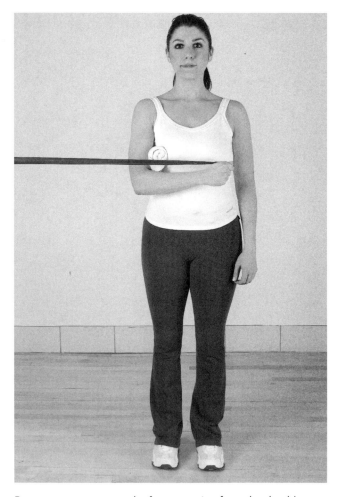

Bent arm moves across the front, rotating from the shoulder.

Lower Trapezius

How do I do this?

1. Lie on your stomach on the floor or a bed, with one arm overhead, elbow straight, thumb pointing up.

2. Raise the working arm straight up, keeping your chest and head down.

3. Return the arm to starting position.

4. Perform seven to ten times with each arm.

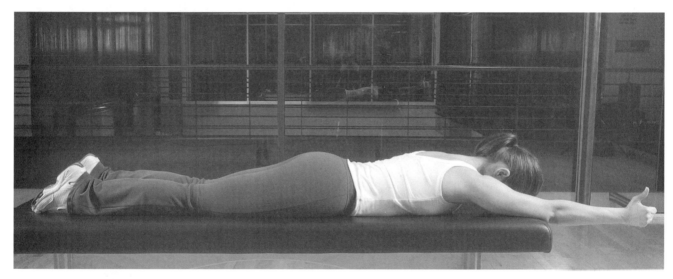

Starting position.

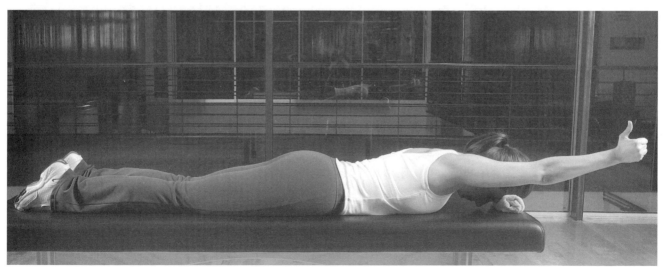

Arm raise.

Extension with Elastic Resistance

How do I do this?

1. Attach an elastic exercise band to the top of a closed door.

2. Stand facing the closed door.

3. Hold the end of the elastic in one hand, with your thumb up.

4. Pull down and back, keeping your elbow straight and close to your side. Pull all the way down so your arm is straight, then slowly return to the starting position.

5. Perform three sets of fifteen, alternating the arms.

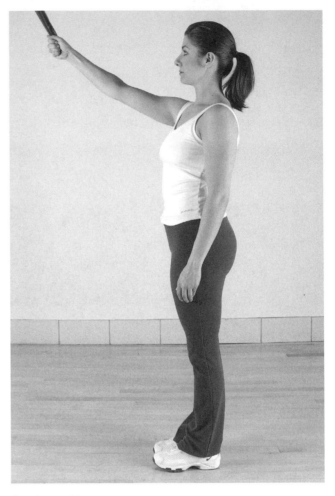

Starting position.

WARM-UP TIP

Try rehearsing the specific movements that you do during your exercise routine or while riding. Sport-specific activity and movement improves coordination, balance, strength, and response time. It also reduces the risk of injury while performing a task if you have prepared your body for the range of motion. If you find you can't complete the specific range of motion of a given exercise without pain, don't do that exercise.

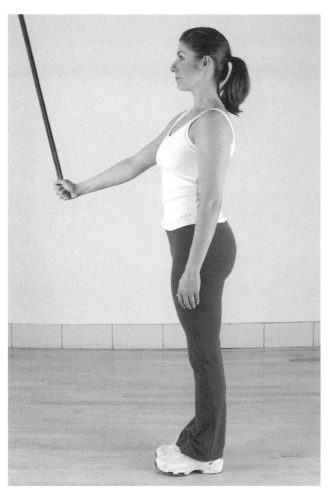

Pull down.

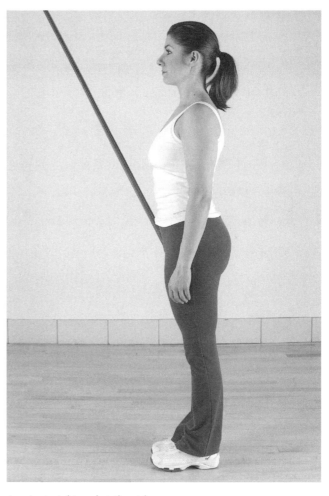

Arm is straight and at the side.

WHY WARM UP?

Warming up can seem like a tedious precursor to the main event but it has lots of important benefits and can make your workout more effective and more enjoyable. Cooling down has many of the same benefits as warming up; it is an important part of any exercise program and one that you should always incorporate into your routine.

Flexion with Elastic Resistance

How do I do this?

1. With your right foot, stand on one end of an elastic exercise band. Hold the other end in your right hand, with your thumb up.

2. Pull the right hand forward and then extend above your shoulders. Keep your arm straight.

3. Slowly return to the starting position.

4. Perform three sets of fifteen on each arm.

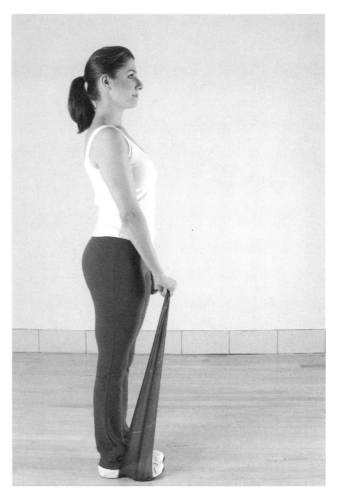

Starting position.

STRETCHING & FLEXIBILITY

The primary reason to stretch is to increase your flexibility. This has an enormous impact on your ability to exercise and to benefit from regular exercise. Increased flexibility will:

• Improve posture and muscle tone
• Enhance coordination
• Improve overall physical well-being
• Reduce stress
• Increase physical efficiency and overall performance
• Reduce the likelihood of injury

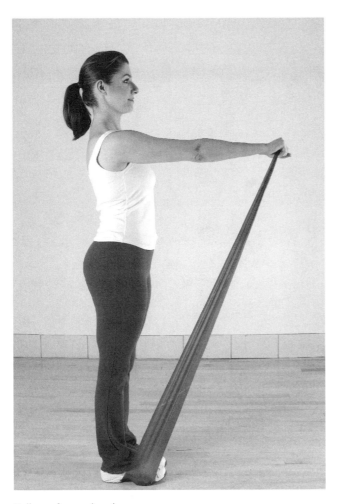

Pull arm forward and up.

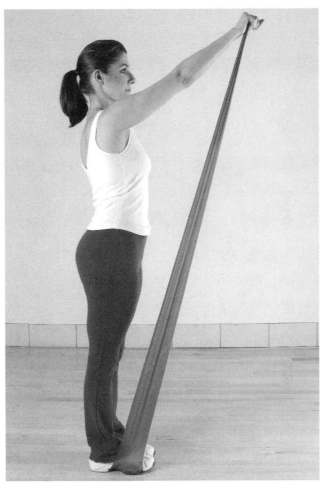

Raise arm overhead.

WARM-UP TIP

Before beginning your exercise routine, try warming up for a few minutes by jogging in place, jumping rope, walking quickly and moving your arms, or any another aerobic activity. This increases circulation and improves muscle performance and flexibility.

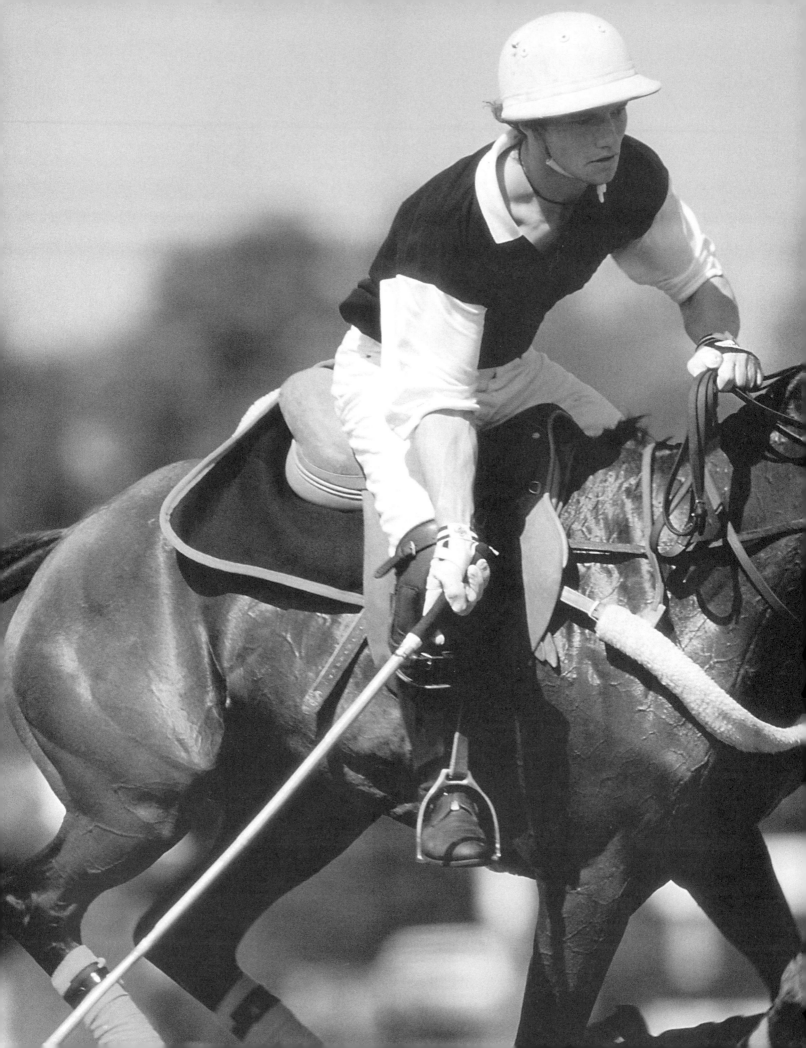

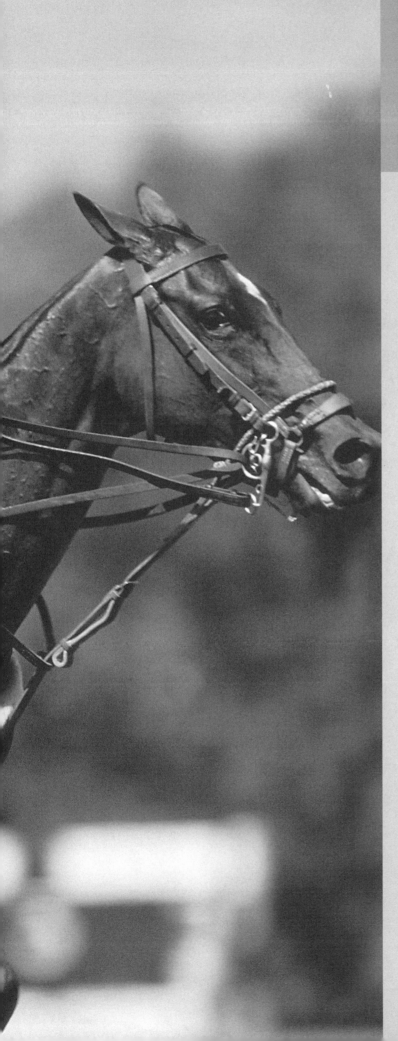

Chapter 2

BALANCE

Balance is one of the keys to successful riding. Good balance and body control are what allow you to achieve "oneness" with your horse. Balance is dynamic; it is dependent upon the movement of your horse, and as such is always changing.

These exercises challenge you to improve your balance. The tilt boards and half-rounds add a measure of complexity to the exercises, and thus more closely mimic the action of your horse. When your balance is automatic and your center of gravity is connected to that of your horse, you will be able to concentrate on the other facets of correct riding.

Correct balance is part of your core stability. When doing these exercises, keep in mind the key elements of core stability:

- Center of gravity
- Stability — absorption of energy
- Power — transmission of energy
- Posture — symmetry
- Movement — asymmetry

Focusing on these elements will help you maintain balance while performing your routines and while riding.

Reciprocal Dumbbell Press

BENEFITS: *Torso control, balance*

Equipment

- Bench
- Dumbbells

How do I do this?

1. Grasp the dumbbells and lie on your back on the bench.

2. Bend your knees and place your feet together on the bench.

3. Push one of the dumbbells upward, extending your arm straight toward the ceiling.

4. As you bring that arm back to the starting position, push the other dumbbell upward. Both arms should be moving simultaneously, in opposite directions.

5. Perform seven to ten repetitions.

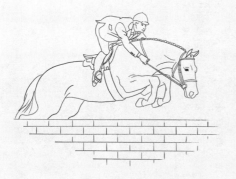

This exercise develops your torso control and balance without the aid of your legs. The alternating movement of the weights creates rotational forces around your torso that must be managed so you remain stable on the bench. This translates to better upper-body/torso position and balance while mounted.

HINTS

- The reciprocal motion of the weights pushes you toward the side of the downward-moving dumbbell.
- Use your torso muscles to stabilize your position on the bench.
- Make sure to pull your shoulder back down onto the bench before lowering the weight.

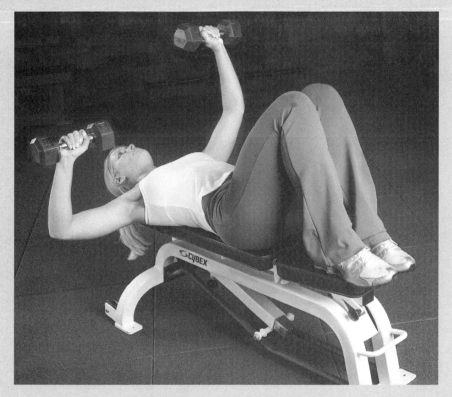

Arms move in opposite directions.

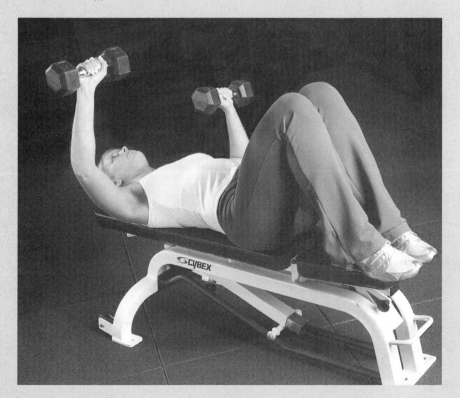

Remain stable and balanced using the torso muscles.

Incline Dumbbell Press with Feet Up

BENEFITS: *Arm and torso efficiency, independence, strength*

Equipment

- Bench
- Dumbbells

How do I do this?

1. Set your bench to an incline of 45 to 60 degrees.

2. Lie on the bench, holding the dumbbells, and pull up your knees so your feet are off the floor.

3. Bring the dumbbells up to shoulder level until your elbows are pointing straight at the floor.

4. Push the weights straight up until your arms are perpendicular to the floor.

5. Return to the starting position, and perform seven to ten repetitions.

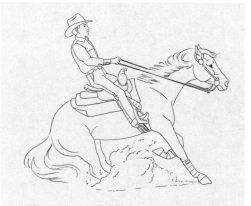

The Incline Dumbbell Press challenges your body's ability to remain steady on the bench; having your feet up makes you less stable. The movement of the weights strengthens your shoulder muscles, helping you to create a more effective riding position while holding the reins.

HINTS

- Be sure to push the weights straight up, away from your chest.
- Keep your back flat on the bench.

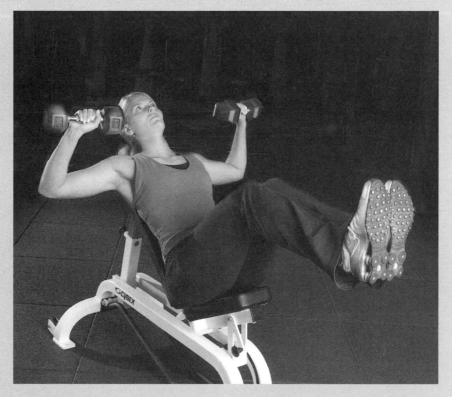

Starting position.

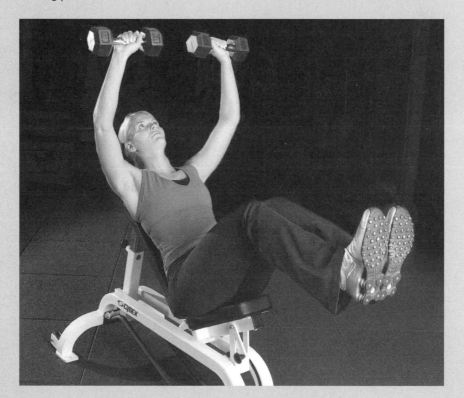

Push arms straight up, legs remaining elevated.

Cable Row in Half-Seat on a Half-Round

BENEFITS: *Stability, balance*

Equipment

- Two 3-foot, half-round foam rollers, pointing straight ahead, shoulder width apart, and 3 feet from the cable or anchor point
- Elastic tubing or cable system, set approximately 5 feet high

How do I do this?

1. Standing carefully on the flat side of the foam rollers, reach forward with one hand and grasp the cable or tubing handle.

2. Assume a half-seat position with your arm extended.

3. Pull the handle toward your torso, bending your arm as you pull.

4. When the handle reaches your torso, extend your arm farther so that your elbow now points behind you.

5. Return to the starting position, then perform seven to ten repetitions before working on the other side.

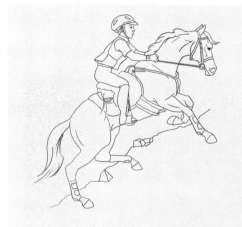

The half-seat position and the tilting half-round foam rollers make this exercise a serious balance challenge. The pull-down movement actually pulls you forward, as if by your mount. Stabilizing against this pull while maintaining balance translates to more effective riding.

CHALLENGE

To make this exercise more challenging, bring the foam rollers closer together.

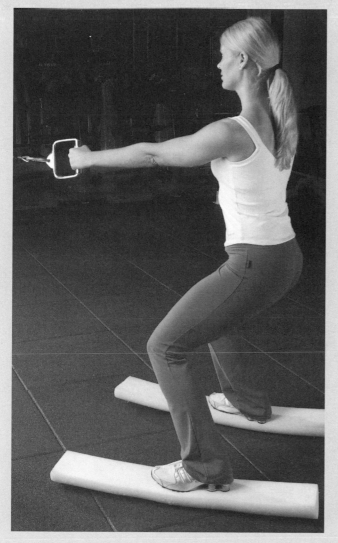

Starting position in a half-seat.

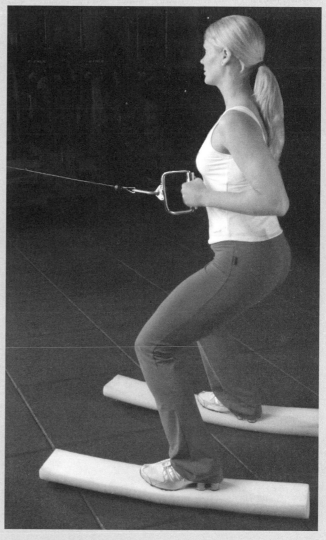

Elbow extends behind torso.

HINTS

- Maintaining your balance while standing on the foam rollers is the key to this exercise.
- Keep your head in a neutral position, with your eyes focused ahead, as if on your horse.
- Keep your back straight.

Half-Seat Cable Row with Two Tilt Boards

BENEFITS: *Balance, stability*

Equipment

- Two tilt boards
- Cable system or elastic tubing with set up T-shaped handle

Setup

- To set the cable height (or anchor point for elastic tubing), assume a half-seat position, then locate your shoulder height. That's the point at which you set your cable.
- Place the tilt boards so they tilt forward and backward. They should be about 4 feet from the anchor point, and your feet about shoulder width apart.

How do I do this?

1. First grasp the handle with both hands, then step onto the tilt boards.

2. After gaining your balance, assume a half-seat position. Your arms should be stretched out in front of you, as if holding the reins.

3. While maintaining a balanced half-seat position, pull the handle straight toward your chest. Pause for 1 second, then return the handle to the starting position.

4. While pulling the handle, pulse up and down, as if performing a modified posting movement.

5. Perform seven to ten repetitions.

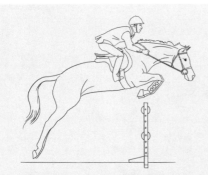

This exercise challenges balance by introducing forward and backward movement into the half-seat position, much like your horse taking off over and landing after obstacles.

CHALLENGE

- Use half-round rollers rather than tilt boards to make the exercise more difficult. Place them flat-side up, so that when you stand on them your feet are across the rollers and you rock back and forth. This is good if you can't hold your half-seat for any length of time.
- You can also place the rollers lengthwise, so that when you stand on them, you rock from side to side. This is especially good if you struggle with your lateral stability.

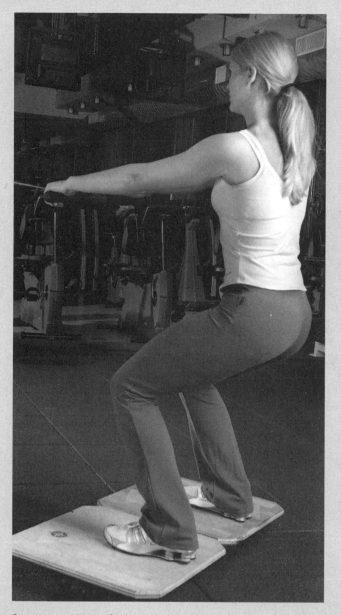

Starting position — find your balance.

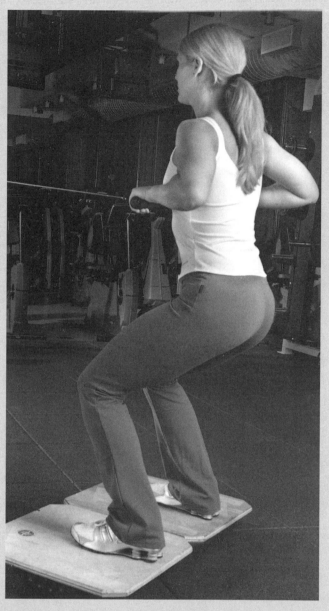

Pull through, maintaining a half-seat position.

HINTS

- Focus on maintaining balance during this movement. When pulling the handle toward you, your body will be pulled forward. Try pushing your hips backward to counteract this force.
- Keep your head in a neutral position with your back flat, your shoulders back, and your eyes up, as if you are mounted.
- This exercise can be done with single tilt board.

Single-Leg Bent-Over Dumbbell Row on Tilt Board

BENEFITS: Single-leg strength, balance

Equipment

- Tilt board, set up so it tilts forward and backward
- Dumbbell

How do I do this?

1. Grasp a dumbbell in one hand, with the arm hanging straight down toward the ground. With your same-side foot, stand on the tilt board and gain your balance.

2. Bend forward from your waist, as if picking up a coin from the ground, and keep the tilt board balanced throughout. You may extend your opposite leg behind you in order to maintain your balance.

3. Keeping your elbow pointed straight back and leading with your elbow, pull the weight straight up until it comes to your side.

4. Slowly lower the weight to the starting position, then perform seven to ten repetitions.

5. Repeat the exercise on the other side.

This very challenging exercise improves balance and stability and strengthens the shoulder muscles in your upper back. Standing on one leg increases the difficulty and allows you to address symmetrical strength in each leg.

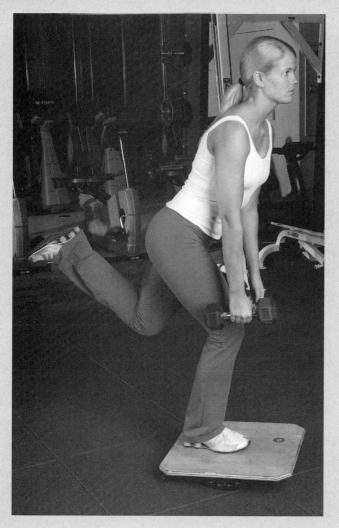

Bend forward with leg extended for balance.

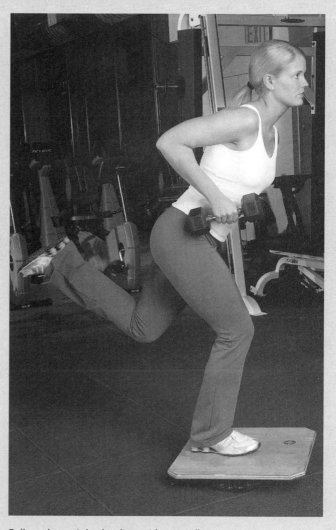

Pull up the weight, leading with your elbow,

HINTS

- Focus on keeping your balance on your supporting leg.
- Keep your back and shoulders straight, with your head and eyes up, as if mounted.

Upright Row on One Leg

BENEFITS: *Shoulder strength, balance, posture*

Equipment

- Two dumbbells

How do I do this?

1. Grasp a dumbbell in each hand and position them together in front of you, below your waist.

2. Shift your weight onto one foot and then lift your other foot from the floor.

3. Without swaying your trunk, pull up the weights directly toward your chin, leading with your elbows. Your elbows should be higher than your shoulders and pointing out to the sides.

4. Pause for 1 second, and then slowly lower the weights to the starting position.

5. Perform seven to ten repetitions, then repeat while standing on the opposite leg.

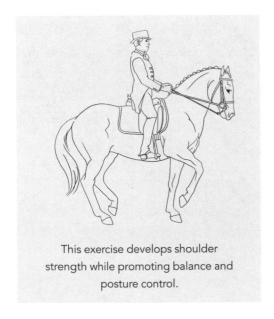

This exercise develops shoulder strength while promoting balance and posture control.

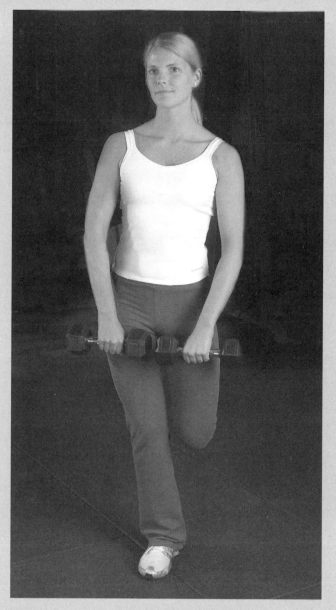

Starting position — weight shifted to one leg.

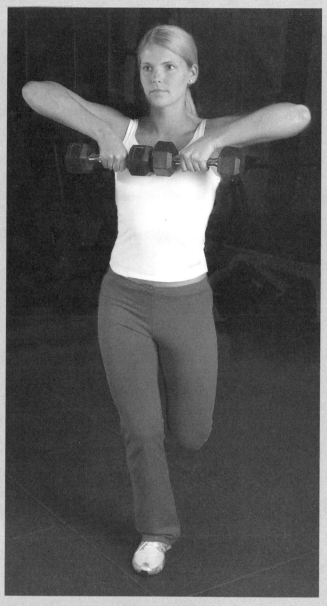

Weights raised, elbows above your shoulders.

HINTS

- Shift your weight on the supporting leg to maintain balance and keep your torso upright.
- Maintain a tall posture throughout this exercise.

Horse-Width Squat on Half-Round

BENEFITS: *Leg strength, lower-body stability, balance*

Equipment

- 3-foot half-round rollers
- Two dumbbells

How do I do this?

1. Grasp a dumbbell in each hand, step on the rollers, and assume a horse-width stance with the dumbbells in front of you. Establish your balance before you continue moving.

2. In one smooth motion, lower yourself toward the floor in a squat, as if to grasp an object at your feet. Your arms should hang straight down. Allow your trunk to bend naturally as you descend, without bending too far forward. Keep your body weight centered over your insteps, not over your heels or the balls of your feet.

3. Keep your balance from tilting inward or outward during the movement, and lower yourself as far as comfort allows.

4. With your legs, push strongly into the ground to return to a standing position.

5. Perform seven to ten repetitions.

The Horse-Width Squat develops leg strength and lower-body stability in a riding position. The half-round foam rollers improve overall stability and balance.

CHALLENGE

Use two 3-foot half-round rollers, set at approximately saddle width with the rollers pointing forward to create a side-to-side roll.

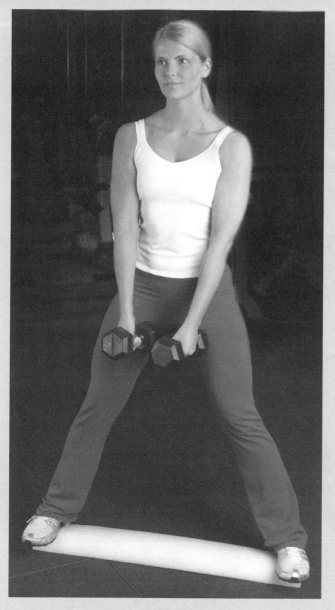

Starting position at horse width.

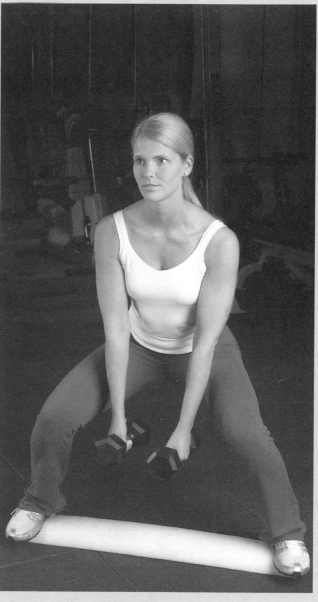

Squat at horse width with dumbbells.

HINTS

- Balance is a critical component of this exercise. Try to remain centered over your insteps at all times.
- You are too far forward if you feel your weight shift from your insteps and the balls of your feet to your toes.
- Keep your head up and eyes facing forward, as if mounted. Keep your trunk long, even as it bends forward.

Unilateral Squat

Benefits: Leg strength, stability

Equipment

- Two dumbbells

How do I do this?

1. Holding a dumbbell in each hand, shift your weight onto one leg, then lift the opposite leg off the floor.

2. In one smooth motion, lower yourself toward the floor in a one-legged squat, as if to grasp an object at your feet. Allow your trunk to bend naturally as you descend, without bending too far forward. You can extend your free leg behind you to help maintain balance. Keep your body weight centered over your supporting instep, not over your heel or the ball of your foot.

3. Lower yourself as far as comfort allows.

4. With your supporting leg, push hard into the ground in order to return to a standing position.

5. Perform seven to ten repetitions, then repeat on the opposite leg.

The Unilateral Squat develops essential independent leg strength for a stable riding position. Performing this exercise on one leg increases the challenge to your equilibrium, further improving your stability in the saddle.

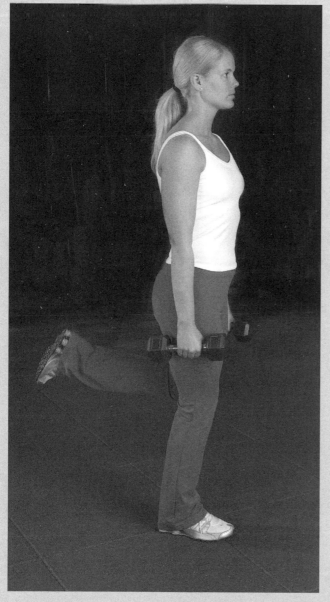

Starting position.

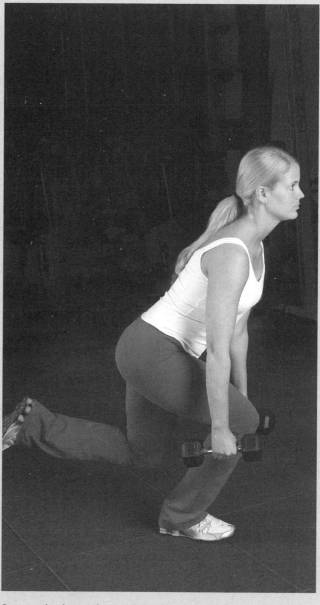

Squat — body weight is centered over the instep.

HINTS

- Balance is a critical component of this exercise. Try to remain centered over your instep at all times.
- You are too far forward if you feel your weight shift from your instep and the ball of your foot to your toes.
- Keep your head up and eyes facing forward, as if mounted.
- Keep your trunk long, even as it bends forward.

Circle Hop

BENEFITS: *Stability, balance, control*

Equipment

- Tape or other marking material, used to mark six points of a circle, approximately 4 feet in diameter, on the floor or mat

How do I do this?

1. Stand on one leg on one of the points. Moving counterclockwise, hop from point to point until you return to the starting position.

2. When landing each hop, be sure to focus on coming to a complete, controlled stop before continuing on to the next point.

3. Perform two counterclockwise and two clockwise revolutions on each leg.

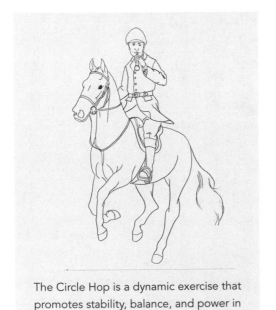

The Circle Hop is a dynamic exercise that promotes stability, balance, and power in the working leg. This will significantly improve a rider's control, particularly when standing in the stirrups.

HINTS

- In order to more effectively maintain balance, try to create more of an upward, rather than lateral, path of movement.
- When landing, try to keep your weight evenly balanced from toe to heel, with you posture straight and eyes forward, as if mounted.

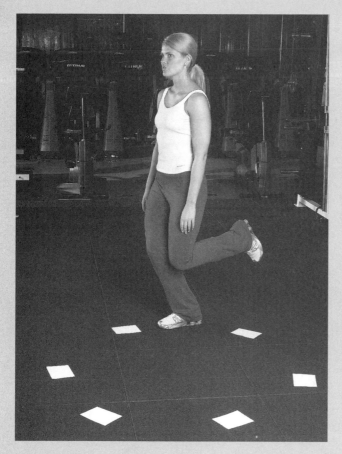

Starting position.

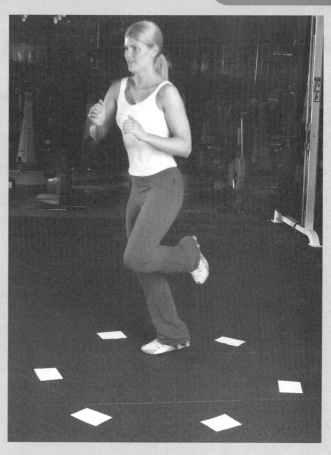

Come to a controlled stop at each point in the circle.

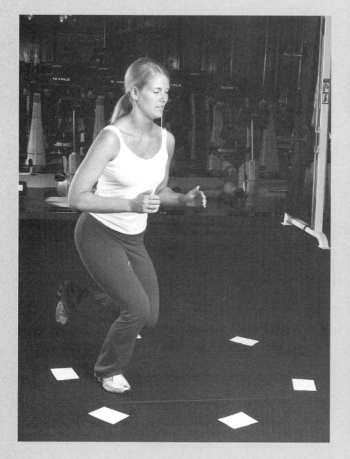

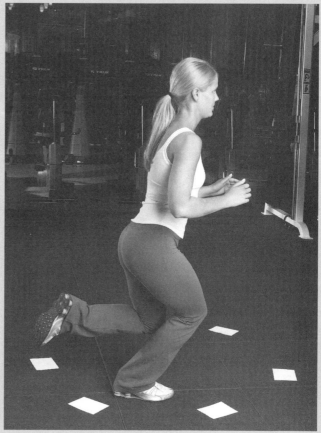

Standing Hip Extension

BENEFITS: *Hip strength, balance, stability*

Equipment

- Cable system or elastic band

How do I do this?

1. Place a cable cuff or loop your elastic band around one ankle. Stand erect, with the anchor point or weight stack in front of you.

2. Take three steps back so that the tube is stretched or the weight stack is elevated slightly.

3. Allow your tethered leg to move forward approximately 2 feet. Remain tall and balanced on your supporting leg.

4. Placing your hands on your hips, remain firm on the supporting leg, keeping its knee slightly bent.

5. Keeping your leg straight, pull the cable behind you and slightly away from your body. Your foot should follow a diagonal path backward and outward, with your toes pointed forward as much as is naturally comfortable. You should have no hip rotation, either in or out.

6. Continue to move the leg as far back and out as possible while still keeping your posture completely upright.

7. Hold the finishing position for 1 second, then return slowly to the starting position.

8. Perform seven to ten repetitions, then repeat the exercise on the other leg.

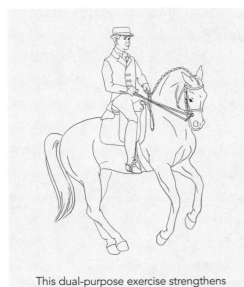

This dual-purpose exercise strengthens and promotes balance around the working hip and improves stability around the supporting hip. The movement is diagonal across the body, replicating both lateral and front-to-back forces that may be experienced in the saddle.

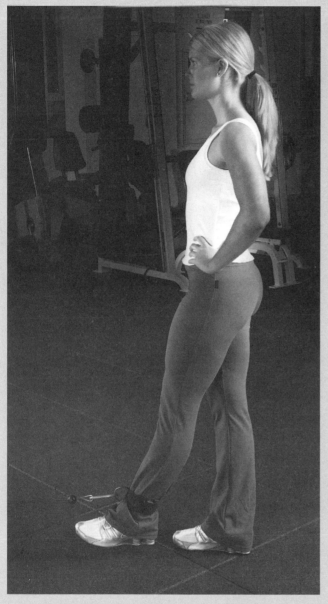

Raise your leg in front of you.

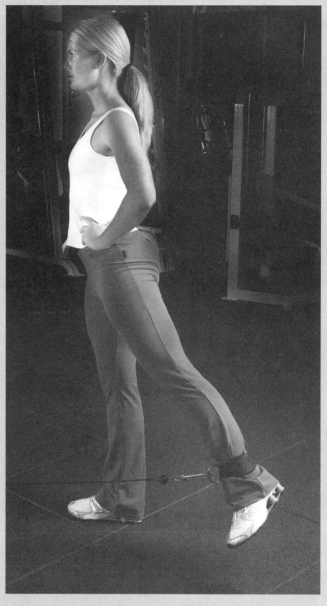

Tethered leg moves behind and out while maintaining upright posture.

HINTS

- Focusing on your supporting leg helps promote stability and control.
- Make sure your hips remain level and pointed forward.
- If this exercise is too difficult at first, hold on to a chair to improve your stability until you are strong enough to do it without support.

Cable Pull-Through with One-Leg Stance

BENEFITS: Balance, hip-muscle control

Equipment

- Cable system or elastic band

How do I do this?

1. Place a cable cuff or loop your elastic band around one ankle. Stand erect with the band's anchor point or the weight stack behind you and slightly closer to your tethered leg.

2. Take three steps forward so that the band is stretched or the weight stack is elevated slightly, with your tethered leg positioned behind you and out to the side. Your entire leg, not just your toes, should be angled slightly away from your body.

3. Keeping your posture tall, shift your body weight onto your supporting leg.

4. Placing your hands on your hips, remain firm on the supporting leg, keeping the knee slightly bent. Remember to keep your hips and body square.

5. Using a pulling motion, pull your tethered leg forward, allowing the knee of the working leg to bend as you pull it forward. Stop when the working leg is pulled up to its highest position possible in front of you.

6. Hold the finishing position for 1 second, then slowly return to the starting position.

7. Perform seven to ten repetitions, then repeat on the other leg.

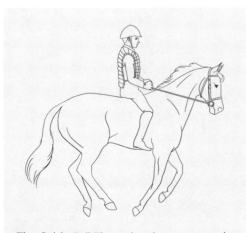

The Cable Pull-Through enhances muscular balance and control around the hip joints.

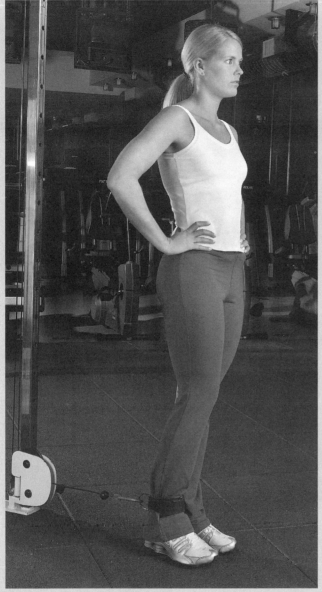

Starting position.

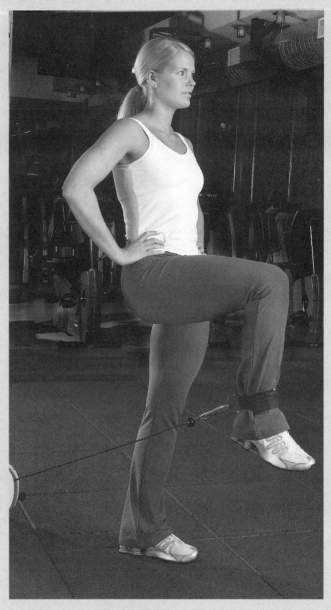

Leg is up, thigh parallel to the floor.

HINTS

- Focusing on the supporting leg will promote stability and control.
- Remember to keep your hips square and steady.
- If this exercise is too difficult at first, hold on to a chair to improve your stability until you are strong enough to complete the exercise without support.

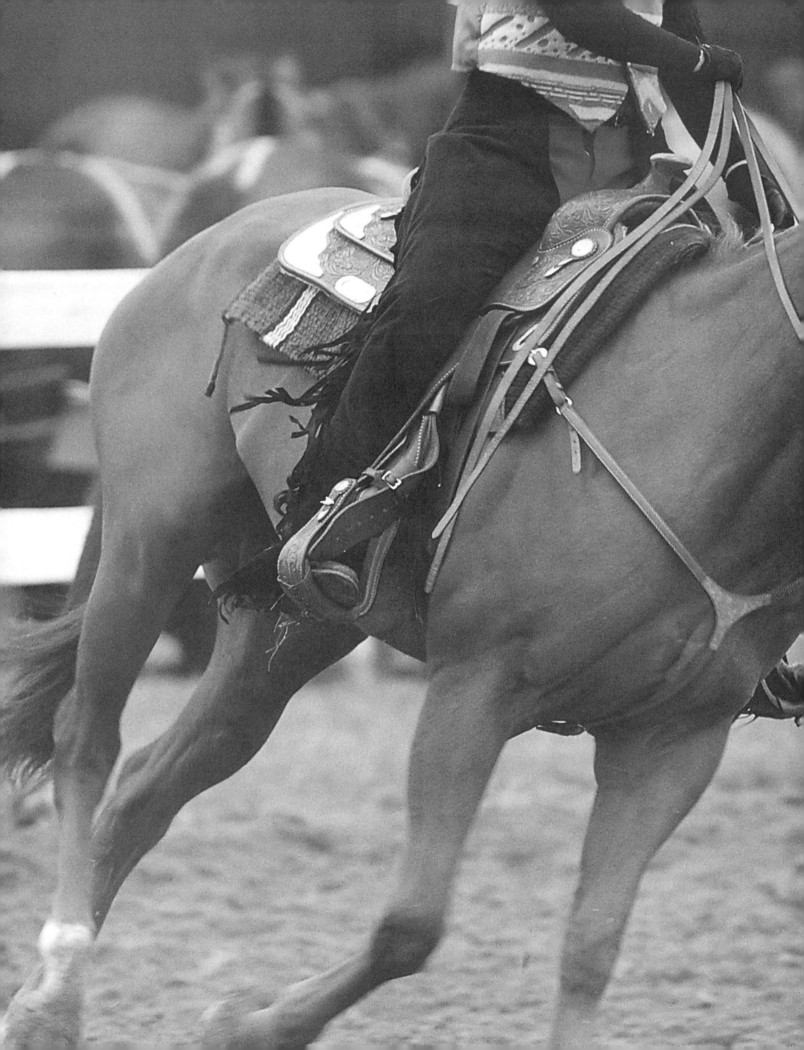

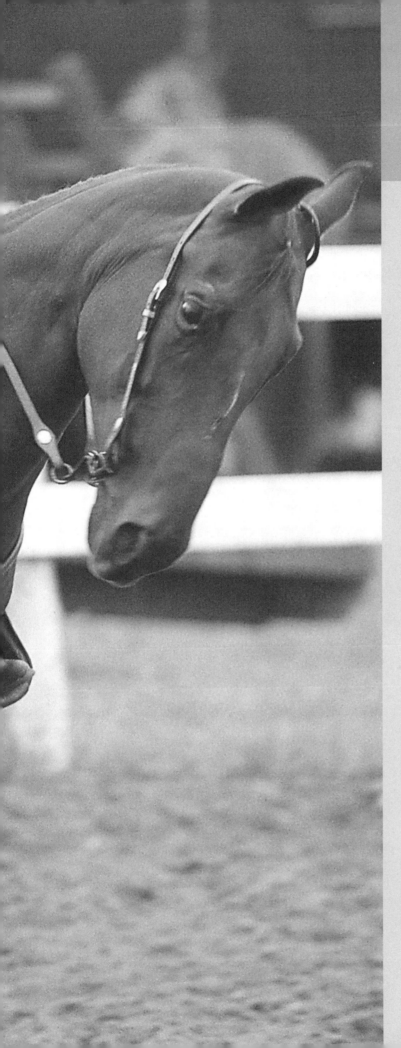

Chapter 3

LOWER BODY

Your legs closely follow your balance as an essential part of your riding foundation. Strong and flexible legs mean your leg position is stable, which in turn contributes to your overall balance. As well as being strong and flexible, your legs need to be independent of each other. Often, your aids will come from one leg while the other remains steady. Your leg should "wrap" around your horse, no matter what your stirrup length.

Your knees and especially your ankles provide shock absorption when you ride, regardless of your gait or discipline. These exercises are an excellent way to prevent injury from the stress caused by riding.

Whether you are new to riding or coming back from a hiatus, the legs are always the sorest part of the body after that first or second ride. They can be a point of tension in the rider, especially the knee and inner upper thigh. These areas are often neglected; performing fitness routines that address them will make your return to the saddle faster and more comfortable.

Squat

BENEFITS: *Leg strength, balance, stability*

Equipment

- Mat
- Dumbbells or wrist weights

How do I do this?

1. Stand up straight with your feet shoulder-width apart. Let your arms hang naturally at your sides.

2. In one smooth motion, lower yourself toward the floor in a squat, as if to grasp an object at your feet. Allow your trunk to bend naturally as you descend. Keep your body weight centered over your insteps.

3. Lower yourself as far as comfort allows.

4. Return to a standing position by pushing hard into the ground with your legs.

5. Perform seven to ten repetitions.

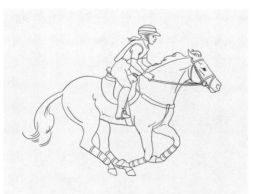

The Squat develops your leg strength, balance, and stability — three fundamentals that help you use your legs effectively while posting, cantering, galloping, or jumping. This exercise also increases your ability to absorb the force of these movements and establish effective body position.

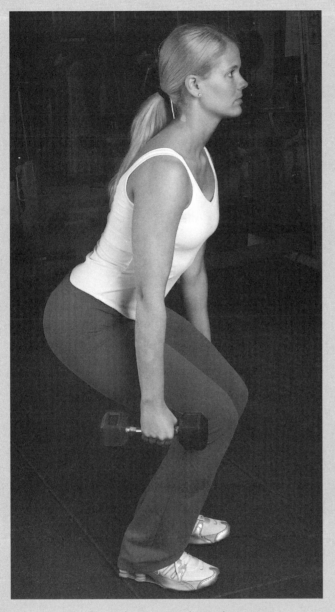

Side view — body weight is centered over the insteps.

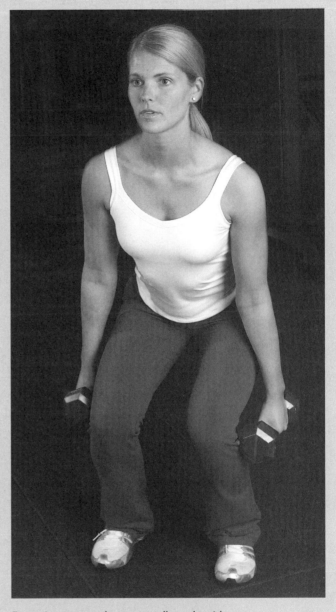

Front view — arms hang naturally at the sides.

HINTS

- Balance is a critical component of this exercise. Remain centered over your insteps at all times.
- Keep your head up and eyes facing forward, as if mounted.
- Allow your trunk to bend forward, but do not round your spine. Maintain a long trunk position even as you bend forward.

Squat at Horse Width

BENEFITS: *Strength, body control*

Equipment

- Mat

How do I do this?

1. Stand up straight with your feet at a width that approximates your leg position in the saddle. Fold your arms across your chest, elbows close to the sides of your body.

2. In one smooth motion, lower yourself toward the floor in a squat, as if to grasp an object at your feet. Allow your trunk to bend naturally as you descend. Keep your body weight centered over your insteps, rather than over your heels or the balls of your feet.

3. Align your knees with the inside of your feet, without pressing them to the outside. Lower yourself as far as comfort allows.

4. With your legs, push hard into the ground to return to a standing position.

5. Perform seven to ten repetitions.

Performing Squats at Horse Width closely mimics your riding position and develops your dynamic strength and body control.

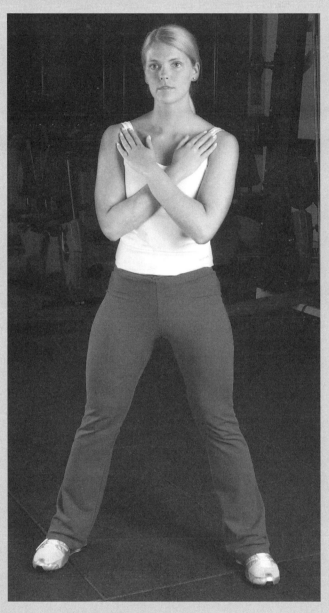

Starting position at horse width.

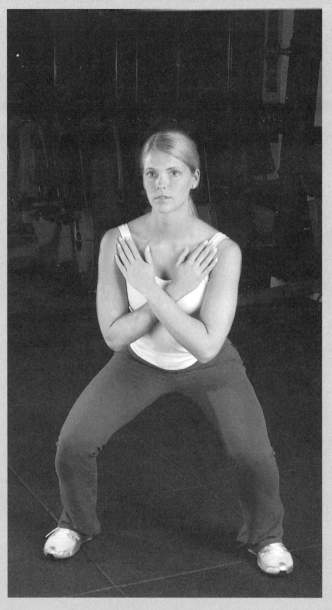

Squat — weight is centered over the insteps.

HINTS

- Balance is a critical component of this exercise. Remain centered over your insteps at all times.
- Keep your head up and eyes facing forward, as if mounted.
- Allow your trunk to bend forward, but do not round your spine. Maintain a long trunk position even as you bend forward.

Squat at Horse Width with Lateral Shift

BENEFITS: *Posture, stability*

Equipment

- Mat

How do I do this?

1. Stand straight with your feet at a width that approximates your position in the saddle. Fold your arms across your chest, elbows close to the sides of your body.

2. In one smooth motion, lower yourself toward the floor in a squat, as if to grasp an object at your feet. Allow your trunk to bend naturally as you descend.

3. Shift your body weight onto one of your legs, keeping both feet in contact with the floor. Keep your body weight centered over your supporting instep, not over your heel or the ball of your foot.

4. Align your knee with the inside of your foot, without allowing it to press to the outside. Lower yourself as far as comfort allows.

5. With your legs, push hard into the ground to return to a standing position. As you approach the standing position, center your weight again and begin the descent into a squat.

6. Perform seven to ten repetitions. Repeat the set with a weight shift onto the other leg.

This version of the Squat challenges the rider through a lateral shift in weight from one leg onto the other. Increased demands on the weighted leg help your postural control and stability.

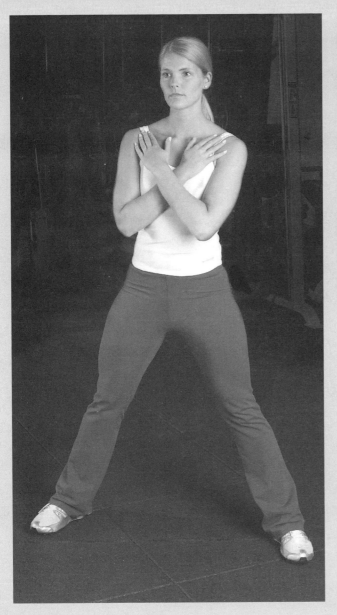

Starting position at horse width.

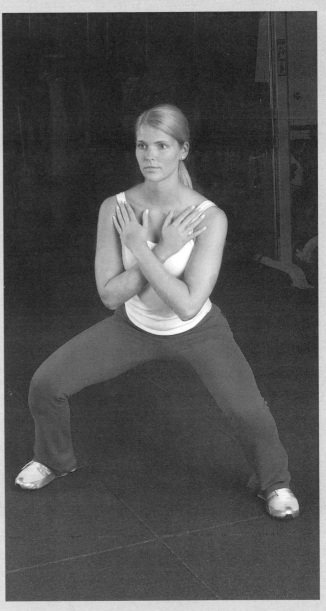

Squat — body weight shifted to right leg.

HINTS

- Try to establish a rhythmic side-to-side motion as your body moves up and down.
- Focus on bringing your body to a stop on each leg as you reach the bottom of the movement.
- Keep your trunk straight and your eyes fixed ahead of you.

Timed Wall Squat with Physioball and Pulsing Motion

BENEFITS: *Leg endurance, posture*

Equipment

- Medium-sized physioball

How do I do this?

1. Stand erect with your back approximately 3 feet in front of a wall, your feet shoulder-width apart.

2. Place a medium-sized physioball behind your pelvis and lower back, leaning into it slightly to keep it pressed against the wall.

3. Begin an up-and-down pulsing movement, allowing your hips and knees to bend only slightly.

4. Perform this movement as long as tolerable, preferably for at least 30 seconds.

5. After a brief rest, repeat the exercise twice.

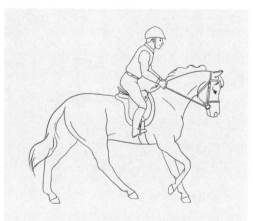

This exercise develops leg endurance and postural stability for your half-seat or galloping position. The pulsing action introduces a small up-and-down motion, which challenges the muscles around the knees and hips. The ball provides instant feedback on weight shift and balance.

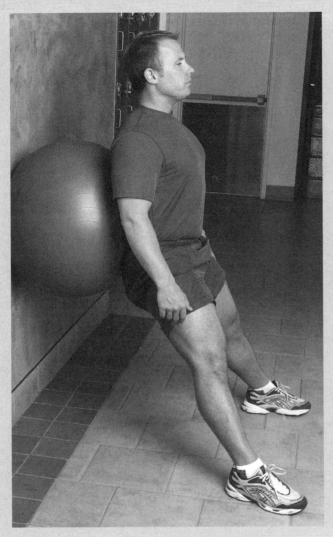

Starting position.

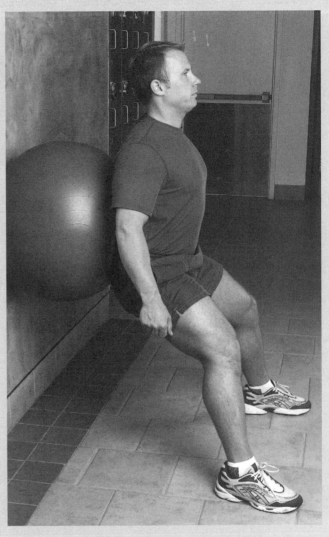

Pulsing with the knees slightly bent.

HINTS

- Try to establish a rhythmic motion that simulates your horse's up-and-down movement.
- Keep your back flat and your shoulders square.
- Pulse faster for an added challenge.

Leg Press at Horse Width

BENEFITS: *Leg strength*

Equipment

- Leg press machine

HINTS

- Move the platform quickly and deliberately in order to generate power.
- Push equally with each leg.

How do I do this?

1. Sit or recline on the bench and position your feet at horse width on the foot platform.

2. Bend your knees comfortably. Press firmly, but not too forcefully, into the platform and locate where in your feet the weight is centered. Move your feet up or down on the platform until you feel the weight align with your insteps.

3. Push the platform deliberately and forcefully until your legs are nearly straightened.

4. Just as deliberately, bring your leg motion to a stop, finishing with your legs fully straightened.

5. Smoothly return to your starting position, coming to a complete stop before attempting the next press. Repeat seven to ten times.

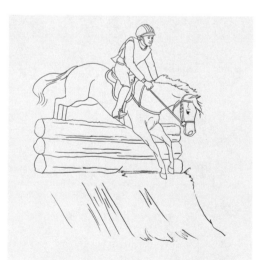

The Leg Press helps you develop the strength necessary to maintain a strong position and manage the forces transmitted to your legs during riding. Because of its stable position, the Leg Press is conducive to increased training loads, which helps build superior leg strength.

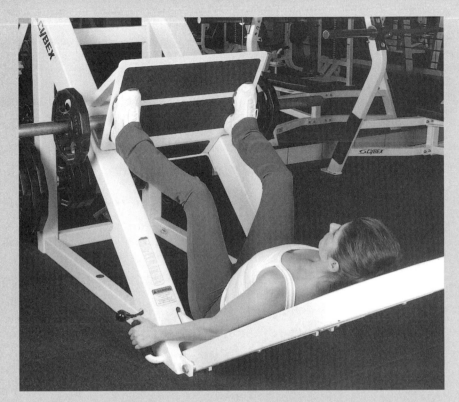

Starting position at horse width.

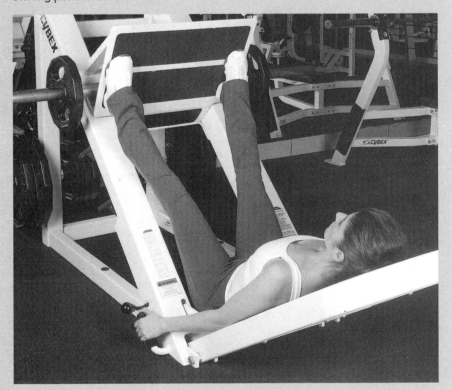

Legs extended.

Step Up

BENEFITS: *Leg strength, stability, balance, posture*

Equipment

- Step or stool 4 to 12 inches (10 to 30 cm) high

How do I do this?

1. Place the step or stool directly in front of you. Place one foot on the middle of the step or stool.

2. Shift your weight forward so that you can feel it align with your instep. Allow your trunk to lean slightly forward in order to complete the shift.

3. Forcefully push down into the step with the supporting leg and move your body up over the step.

4. Come to a standing position with both feet on the step.

5. Leaving the supporting foot on the step, lower your body, in a controlled manner, back to the starting position.

6. Perform seven to ten repetitions on one leg, then repeat with the other.

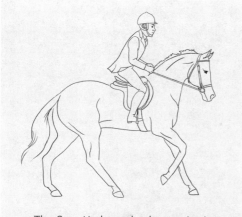

The Step Up lower-body exercise is essential to the development of your leg strength. Because the exercise is done on one leg at a time, it promotes stability, balance, and postural control.

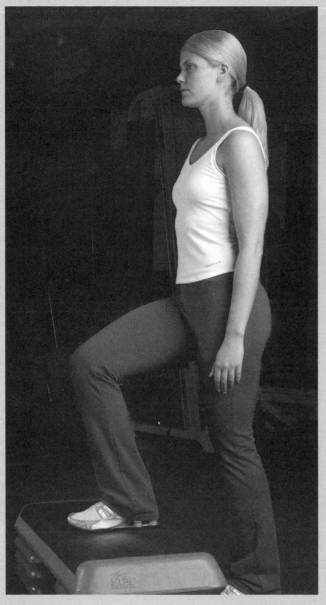

Starting position.

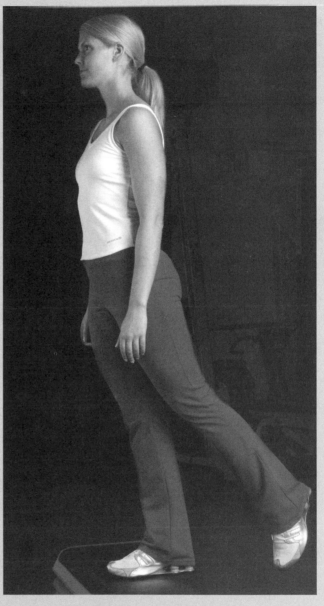

Come into a standing position, bringing both feet onto the step.

HINTS

- Beginning the exercise with your weight directly over the supporting foot is critical to success.
- Keep your supporting knee aligned with the middle of your foot throughout the exercise.
- Use the muscles in your supporting leg to pull yourself up. If you find yourself pushing with the other leg, lower the step height.

Anterio-Lateral Step Up

BENEFITS: *Stability, leg strength*

Equipment

- Step or stool 4 to 12 inches (10 to 30 cm) high

How do I do this?

1. Place a step or stool in front of and about 2 feet to the outside of one of your legs.

2. Place your foot on the middle of the step or stool so that your leg is angled approximately 45 degrees in front and to the side of your body.

3. Shift forward and sideways so that you can feel your body weight align with the instep of your foot. Remain facing forward, keeping your body straight. Allow your trunk to lean slightly forward in order to complete the weight shift.

4. Forcefully push down into the step with that leg and move your body up over the step.

5. Come to a standing position with both feet on the step. Keep your hands at your side, shoulders relaxed.

6. Leaving the supporting foot on the step, slowly lower your body to the starting position.

7. Perform seven to ten repetitions, then repeat with your other leg.

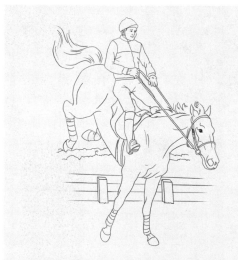

The Anterio-Lateral Step Up presents the same challenges as the Step Up with the added difficulty of having to move your body in a horizontal path. Though this motion does not regularly occur during riding, the action of the working leg helps promote stability and keeps the leg from moving away from your body (as if the stirrups were swinging outward).

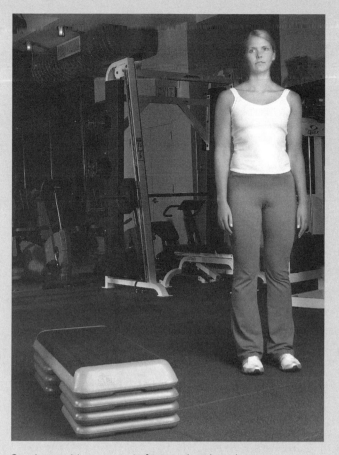

Starting position — step in front and to the side.

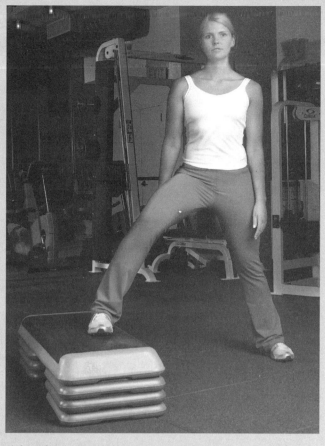

Shifting forward and sideways toward the step.

HINTS

- Remain facing forward without rotating your trunk or hips.
- Pull hard with your leg in order to move your body horizontally.
- Keep your weight over your supporting foot.

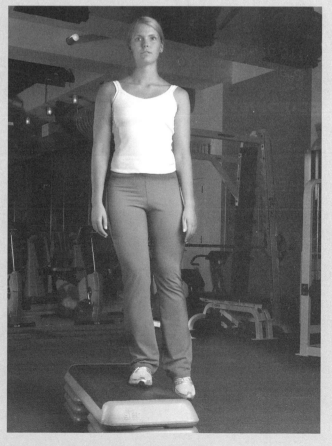

Come to a standing position, with both feet on step.

Lateral Step Up

BENEFITS: Hip and leg stability

Equipment

- Step or stool 4 to 12 inches (10 to 30 cm) high

How do I do this?

1. Place a step or stool approximately 2 feet to the side of one of your legs.

2. Place your foot on the middle of the step or stool so that your legs are slightly more than horse-width apart.

3. Shift your weight onto the foot on the step so that you can feel it align with your instep. Remain facing forward, keeping your body straight. Allow your trunk to lean forward slightly to maintain balance.

4. Forcefully push down into the step with the supporting leg and move your body up over the step.

5. Come to a standing position with both feet on the step. Keep your hands at your sides, shoulders relaxed.

6. Leaving the supporting foot on the step, slowly lower your body to the starting position.

7. Perform seven to ten repetitions, then repeat with the other leg.

The Lateral Step Up is a strength-building exercise that will help you maintain a more stable position in the saddle. Pulling the body laterally ensures that the hips can continue to "squeeze" effectively, making the rider more efficient.

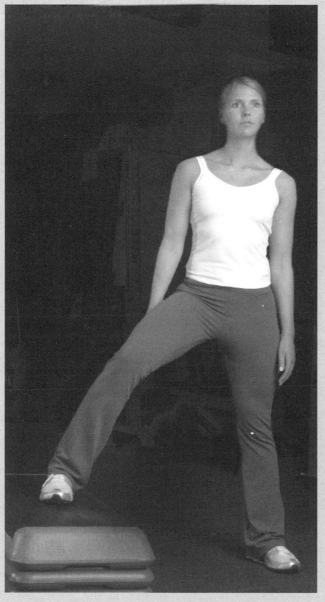

Leg extended to the step.

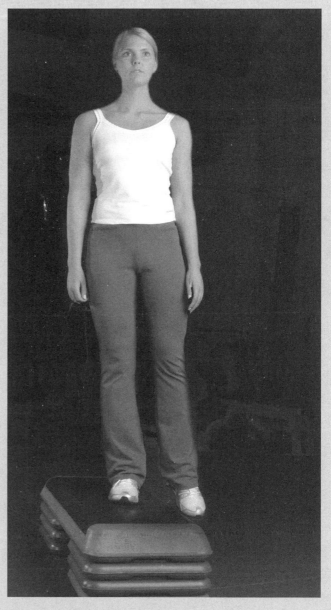

Coming into the standing position on the step.

HINTS

- Remain facing forward; do not rotate your trunk or hips.
- Pull hard with your leg in order to move your body horizontally.
- Keep your weight over your supporting foot.

Lunge

BENEFIT: *Force absorption*

Equipment

- Mat

CHALLENGE

Add dumbbells or wrist weights to this exercise.

How do I do this?

1. Standing tall on a mat, focus on a spot on the floor approximately 3 feet in front of your body.

2. Shifting your weight forward, take an exaggerated step toward that spot, with your whole body moving forward as a single unit.

3. Land on your heel, then quickly transfer weight onto your whole foot, sinking your body onto your front, working leg.

4. Descend to a comfortable lunge position, then bring your body to a complete stop.

5. Forcefully push down and forward with the front leg to push back to the starting position.

6. Repeat with the opposite leg; then, in an alternating fashion, perform a series of seven to ten repetitions on each leg.

The Lunge builds force-absorbing and force-producing capabilities in your legs, giving you greater control, particularly when landing over obstacles.

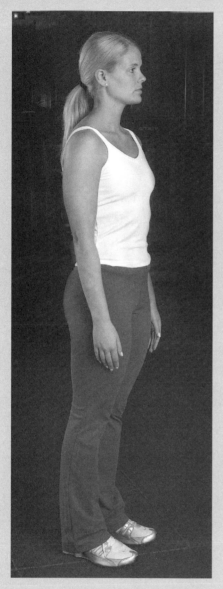

Starting stance.

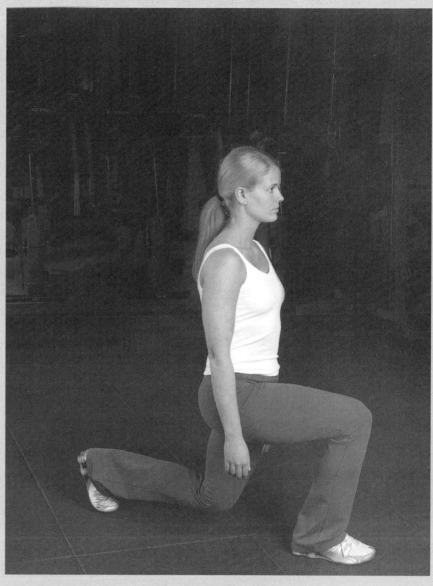

Completed lunge.

HINTS

- When landing on the working foot, allow your trunk to lean forward slightly until you feel your body weight shift to the middle of your foot. Be sure to keep your heel on the floor.
- Concentrate on using only your legs, keeping your trunk and arms quiet during the movement.
- Use a starting mark on the floor and always return to that mark. This will ensure adequate force production.

Crossover Lunge

BENEFIT: Lateral stability

Equipment

- Mat

How do I do this?

1. Select a spot on the floor approximately 1 foot in front and 2 feet to the side of your body.

2. Shift your weight forward and take an exaggerated step toward the spot with the opposite leg, moving your whole body forward and laterally as a single unit.

3. Land on your heel, then quickly transfer the weight onto your whole foot and sink onto your front leg.

4. Descend to a comfortable lunge position, then bring your body to a complete stop.

5. Forcefully push down, forward, and slightly to the side with the front leg to push back to the starting position.

6. Repeat with the opposite leg, then alternate, performing a series of seven to ten repetitions with each leg.

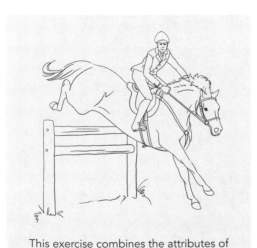

This exercise combines the attributes of the Lunge and the Lateral Step Up, promoting force production and absorption while creating lateral stability.

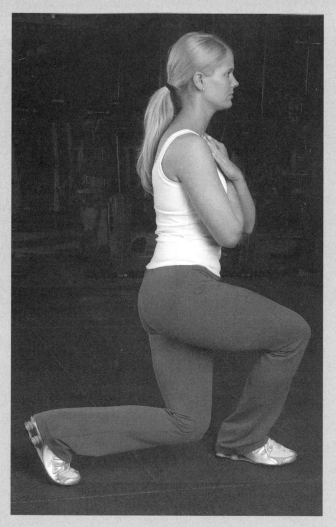

Crossover lunge — side view.

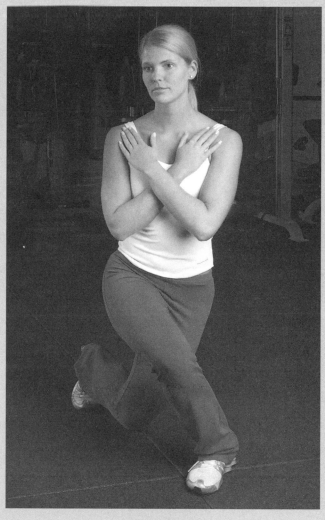

Crossover lunge — front view.

HINTS

- Be sure to keep your feet and chest facing straight forward, as if riding, rather than toward the target on the floor.
- When landing on the lead foot, allow your trunk to lean forward slightly and to the side until you feel your body weight shift to the middle of your foot. Be sure to keep your heel and the flat of your foot firmly on the floor.
- Use only your legs. Concentrate on keeping your trunk and arms quiet during the movement.
- Use a starting mark on the floor. Always return to the mark. This will ensure adequate force production.

Forward Leg Swing

BENEFITS: *Leg independence and stability*

Equipment

- Cable system or elastic band

How do I do this?

1. Place a cable cuff or loop your elastic band around one ankle. Stand erect, facing away from the band's attachment or weight stack.

2. Take two steps forward so that the band is stretched behind you or the weight stack is elevated slightly.

3. Allow the working leg to move backward and slightly to the outside. Bend your knee slightly as your leg moves backward.

4. Placing your hands on your hips, remain firm on your supporting leg. Keep the supporting knee slightly bent and continue to face forward. Do not allow your body to rotate toward the working leg.

5. Using a sweeping motion, pull the working leg forward, first moving at the hip, then completing the motion by straightening the knee.

6. Hold the finishing position for 1 second, then slowly return to the starting position.

7. Perform a series of seven to ten repetitions, then repeat on the other leg.

This exercise has a dual function: While one leg stabilizes your body, the other leg moves. The combination helps improve stability on the supporting leg, translating to increased control in the saddle, particularly during turns.

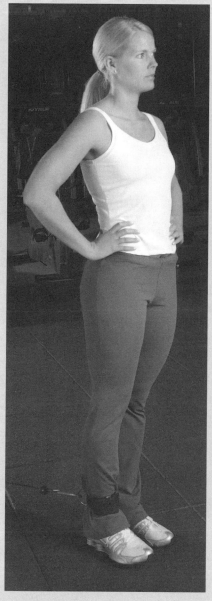

Starting stance.

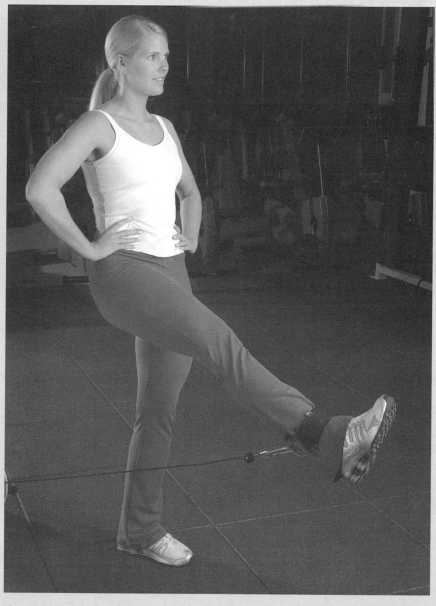

The working leg is forward and straight.

HINTS

- Focus on the supporting leg. This promotes stability and control.
- Keep your hips stable and square.
- If this exercise is too difficult at first, hold on to a chair to help stabilize yourself until you are strong enough to do the exercise without support.

Standing Hip Extension with External Rotation

BENEFITS: *Hip strength and coordination, stability*

Equipment

- Cable system or elastic band

How do I do this?

1. Place a cable cuff or loop your elastic band around one ankle. Stand erect with the band's anchor point or weight stack in front you and slightly closer to your tethered (working) leg.

2. Take three steps backward so that the band is stretched or the weight stack is elevated slightly. Your working leg should be positioned in front of you. Your posture should be tall with your body weight shifted onto your supporting leg.

3. Place your hands on your hips and remain firm on the supporting leg, keeping its knee slightly bent.

4. Pull the working leg straight backward, keeping the knee straight.

5. After the working leg moves behind the supporting leg, rotate your body in the direction of the working leg, keeping the supporting leg fixed in place.

6. Maintain your balance during this movement and stop when you are turned to the side.

7. Hold the finish position for 1 second, then return slowly to the starting position.

8. Perform a series of seven to ten repetitions and repeat with the other leg.

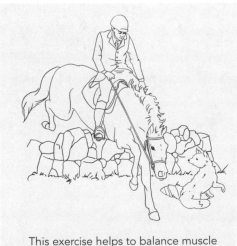

This exercise helps to balance muscle strength and coordination around the hip joints, improving their stability and, therefore, movement control in the saddle.

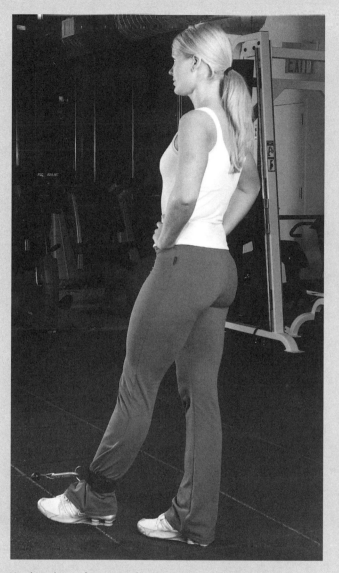

Working leg in front, weight is on your supporting leg (step 2).

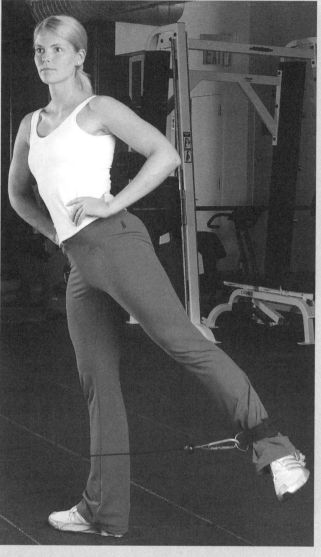

Rotate in the direction of your working leg (step 5).

HINTS

- Focus on the standing leg in order to promote stability and control.
- If this exercise is too difficult at first, hold on to a chair to improve stability until you are strong enough to do the exercise without support.

Hip Abduction

BENEFIT: *Lateral stability*

Equipment

- Cable system or elastic band

How do I do this?

1. Stand erect with your side to weight stack or band's anchor point. Attach cuff to the ankle farther from the stack.

2. Take two steps to the side so that the band is stretched or the weight stack is elevated slightly.

3. Position the tethered (working) leg next to your supporting leg. Your posture should be tall and balanced.

4. Placing your hands on your hips, remain firm on the supporting leg, keeping its knee slightly bent. Lift your working leg and cross it in front of the supporting leg. Do not allow your body to rotate toward or away from the working leg.

5. Using a sweeping motion, push the working leg to the side, away from your body. Continue as far as possible without leaning to the side.

6. Hold the finishing position for 1 second, then slowly return to the starting position.

7. Perform a series of seven to ten repetitions, then repeat on the other leg.

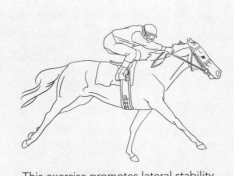

This exercise promotes lateral stability, and when used in conjunction with Hip Adduction (page 92) creates muscular and functional balance around your hip joints and feet.

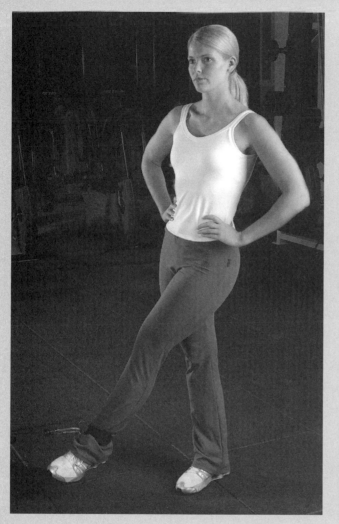

The working leg crosses in front of the supporting leg.

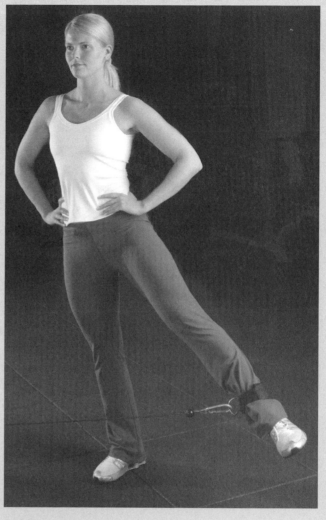

Push the working leg out to the side.

HINTS

- Focus on the supporting leg. This promotes stability and control.
- Keep your hips stable and square.
- If this exercise is too difficult at first, hold on to a chair to stabilize yourself until you are strong enough to do the exercise without support.

Hip Adduction

BENEFIT: *Lateral stability*

Equipment

- Cable system or elastic band

How do I do this?

1. Place a cable cuff or loop elastic band around one ankle. Stand erect with the band's attachment or weight stack to your side, next to your tethered (working) leg.

2. Take two steps to the side of your working leg so that the band is stretched or the weight stack is elevated slightly. Your legs should be approximately horse-width apart.

3. Stand square and tall with your body weight shifted onto your supporting leg. Lift the tethered (working) leg off the ground.

4. Placing your hands on your hips, remain firm on the leg without the cuff, keeping the knee slightly bent.

5. Using a sweeping motion, pull the working leg toward the supporting leg. Stop when the working leg crosses your supporting leg.

6. Hold the finishing position for 1 second, then slowly return to the starting position.

7. Perform a series of seven to ten repetitions, then repeat on the other leg.

This exercise promotes your lateral stability, and when used in conjunction with Hip Abduction (page 90) creates muscular and functional balance around the hip joints and feet.

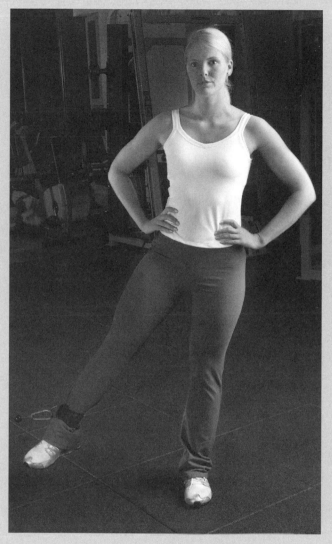

Body weight is centered on the supporting leg.

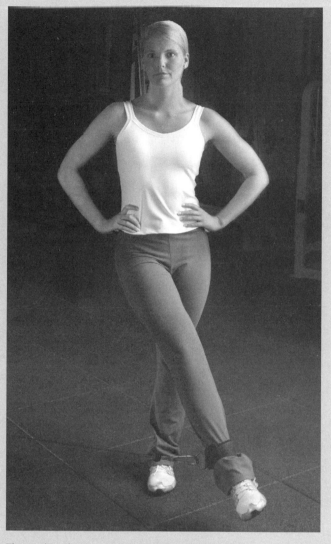

The working leg crosses in front, keeping hips even.

HINTS

- Focus on the standing leg. This promotes stability and control.
- Keep your hips stable and square.
- If this exercise is too difficult at first, hold on to a chair to help stabilize yourself until you are strong enough to do the exercise without support.

Straight-Knee Dead Lift

BENEFITS: *Hip extensor strength and hamstrings*

Equipment

- Mat
- Weight bar or dumbbells

How do I do this?

1. Stand erect with your feet at a width that approximates your position in the saddle. Hold the weight bar in front of you. If you are using dumbbells, let your arms fall naturally at your sides.

2. Keeping your back straight, push your hips backward, allowing your trunk to bend forward from the hips. Stop when you can no longer push your hips backward.

3. Return to standing position.

4. Repeat seven to ten times.

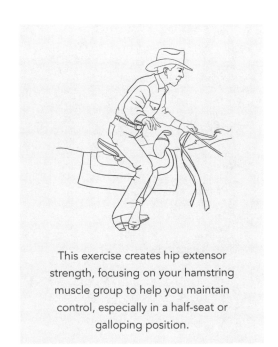

This exercise creates hip extensor strength, focusing on your hamstring muscle group to help you maintain control, especially in a half-seat or galloping position.

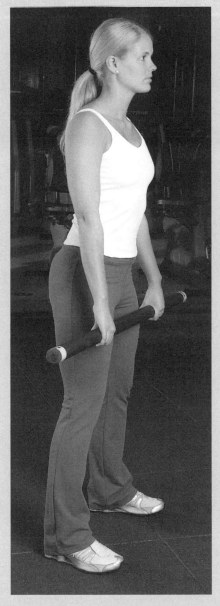

Starting stance.

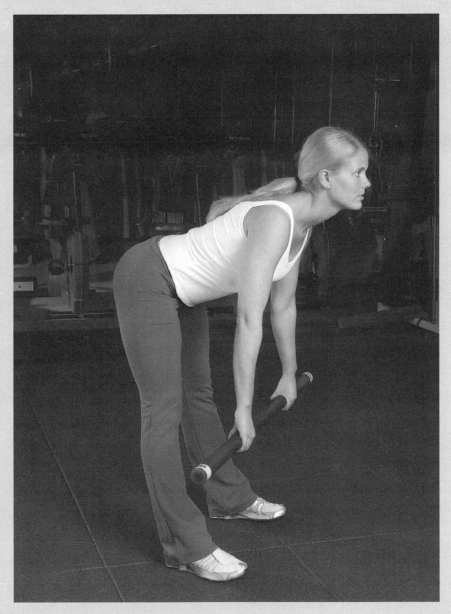

Pushing backward from the hips.

HINTS

- The object is to push the hips back but not reach the floor. Stop when you feel tension in the backs of your thighs.
- Keep your back straight; do not round your shoulders or spine.
- Keep your weight centered over your feet at all times; do not shift onto the balls of your feet or your toes.

Bent-Knee Dead Lift

BENEFIT: *Hip extensor strength and gluteals*

Equipment

- Mat
- Weight bar or dumbbells

How do I do this?

1. Stand erect with your feet at a width that approximates your position in the saddle. Hold the weight bar in front of you. If you are using dumbbells or wrist weights, allow your arms to rest naturally at your sides.

2. Bend your knees slightly.

3. Keeping your back straight, push your hips backward, allowing your trunk to bend forward from the hips. Stop when you can no longer push your hips backward.

4. Return to standing position.

5. Repeat seven to ten times.

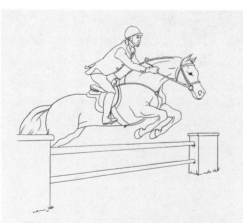

This exercise strengthens your extensor muscles, focusing on your larger gluteal muscles rather than the hamstrings. The gluteals are large hip muscles that provide power and control and are essential during all facets of riding, especially posting and jumping.

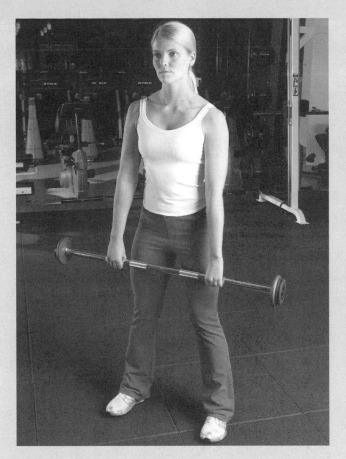

Starting position.

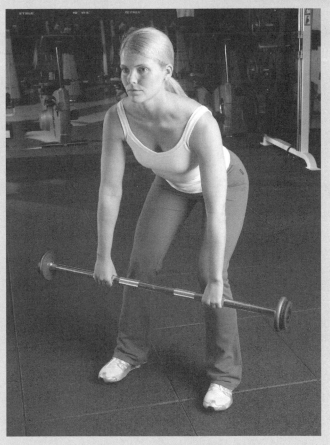

Bending from the hips with the knees slightly bent.

HINTS

- The object is to push the hips back but not reach the floor. Stop when you feel tension in the backs of your thighs.
- Keep your back straight; do not round your spine or shoulders.
- Keep your weight centered over your feet at all times; do not shift onto the balls of your feet or your toes.

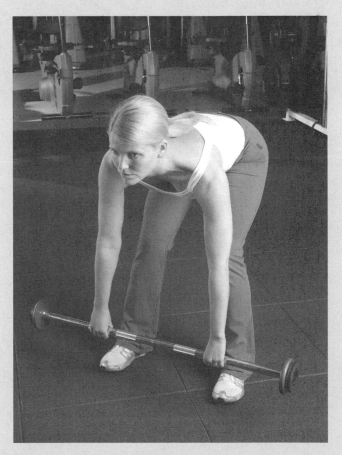

The back is straight and the hips are pushed backward.

Leg Extension

BENEFIT: *Knee strength*

Equipment

- Leg-extension machine, ankle weights, or elastic tubing (a tall chair or counter works when a leg-extension machine is not available)

How do I do this?

1. Assume a seated position in the leg-extension machine. Keep your thighs parallel to the floor, your back upright, and your legs free to move from the knees. If you are using tubing, sit on a chair or the edge of a table. Secure one end of the tubing to the chair or table leg and the other end to your ankle. You can shorten or lengthen the tubing to adjust the resistance.

2. Working one leg at a time, extend the leg fully, so that it is pointing straight away from you.

3. Slowly bend your knee, lowering your foot approximately 12 inches. Pause for 1 second, then return to the extended position.

4. Perform seven to ten repetitions, then repeat with other leg.

HINTS

- Keep your hips firmly on the seat.
- If you are using bands or elastic tubing, tie one end to the chair leg and the other to your ankle — make the band tight enough to provide resistance. If you are using ankle weights, you can increase the weights or the velocity of the exercise.

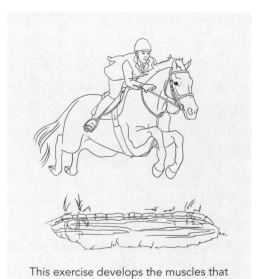

This exercise develops the muscles that control movement around the knee and are needed for posting, jumping, half-seat, and full galloping positions.

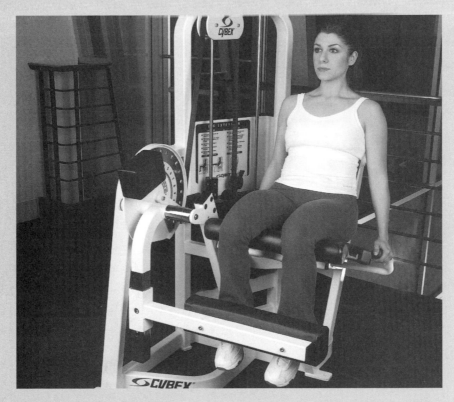

Starting position.

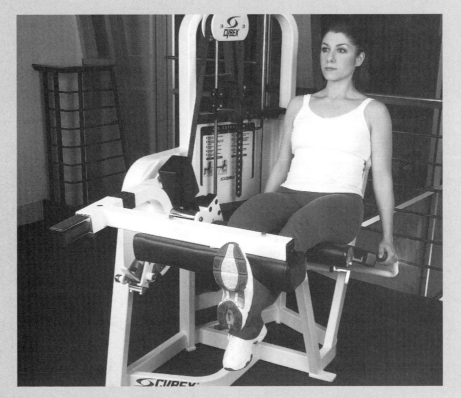

Working leg is fully extended.

Seated Leg Curl

BENEFIT: *Hamstring strength*

Equipment

- Seated leg-curl machine or table and elastic tubing

How do I do this?

1. Sit on the leg-curl machine with both legs extended. If you are using elastic tubing, sit on the edge of a table with one leg extended. Secure one end of the tubing to your ankle and the other to a point in front of you at approximately the same height as the table. The tubing should be stretched slightly and offer resistance when you lower the leg.

2. Pull one of your extended legs downward, bending the knee as far as possible.

3. Hold the bent position for 1 second, then slowly return to the extended position.

4. Perform seven to ten repetitions, then repeat with the other leg.

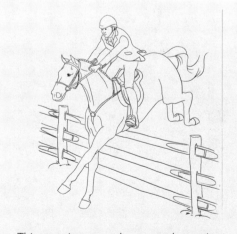

This exercise strengthens your hamstring muscles where they intersect in the knee joint. Strength in this area is vitally important for landing after obstacles.

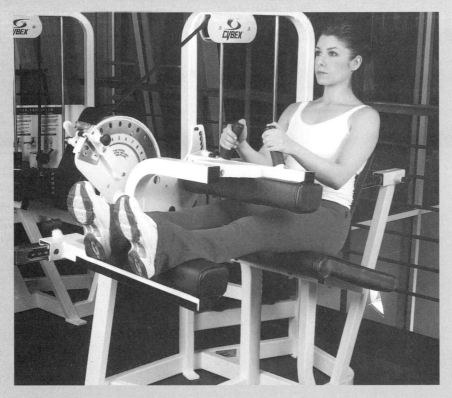

Starting position.

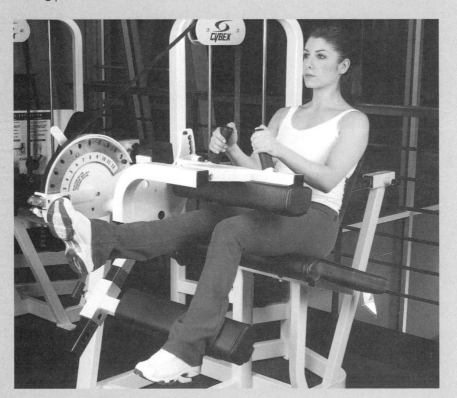

Right leg is extended while left leg pushes down, bending at the knee.

Standing Heel Raise at Horse Width with Angulation

BENEFITS: Calf strength, ankle flexibility

Equipment

- Exercise step, block, or 2 x 4

CHALLENGE

Increase the difficulty of this exercise by using hand weights.

How do I do this?

1. Stand erect with your feet approximately horse-width apart. Your knees should be slightly wider than shoulder width.

2. Place the balls of your feet on the step so that your heels are lifted off the ground.

3. Slowly drop your heels to the ground and hold for a couple of seconds.

4. Rise back up on your toes as high as possible while still maintaining your balance.

5. As you rise, pull your knees toward each other, stopping when they are just inside shoulder width.

6. Slowly return your heels and knees to the starting position.

7. Perform seven to ten repetitions.

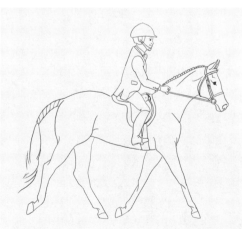

This exercise strengthens your calf muscles and improves your ability to generate force through your ankles and feet in a riding position, while shifting your weight from foot to foot. These muscles play an important role in controlling your body position on the horse.

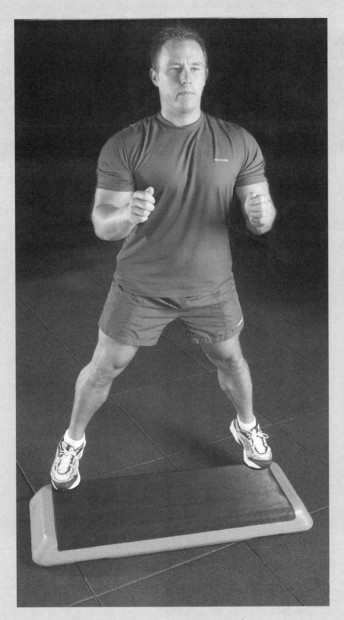

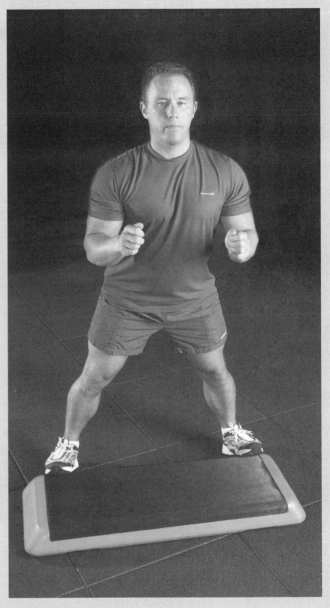

Balls of the feet are on the step — heels raised.

Pressing the heels to the floor.

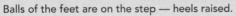

HINTS

- Create a fluid movement without bouncing.
- Stand square and look straight ahead, as if you are riding.

Seated Heel Raise at Horse Width

BENEFIT: *Ankle control*

Equipment

- Seated heel-raise device or elastic tubing and block

HINT

- Keep your body upright, with your head up and eyes forward, as if mounted.

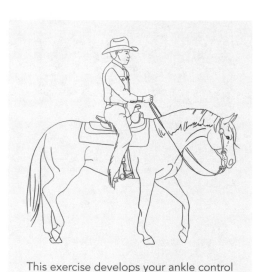

This exercise develops your ankle control when the knee is flexed. Because your ankles act as shock absorbers, they need to be both strong and flexible. This will also help prevent injuries to your feet, ankles, and knees.

How do I do this?

1. Sit on the heel-raise device with your knees under the pads, or select a stool or chair on which you can sit with your thighs parallel to the ground and tie a large loop in the elastic tubing.

2. Position your feet at horse width and place the balls of your feet on the steps or a block.

3. If you are using elastic tubing, place one end of the elastic loop under the balls of your feet and bring the opposite end up and over your knees, making sure not to cover your kneecaps. The elastic should be slightly stretched and snug.

4. Sit up straight, then raise your heels off the floor as high as possible.

5. Hold for 1 second, then lower to starting position.

6. Drop your heels as low as possible. Hold for 1 second, then return to starting position.

7. Perform seven to ten repetitions.

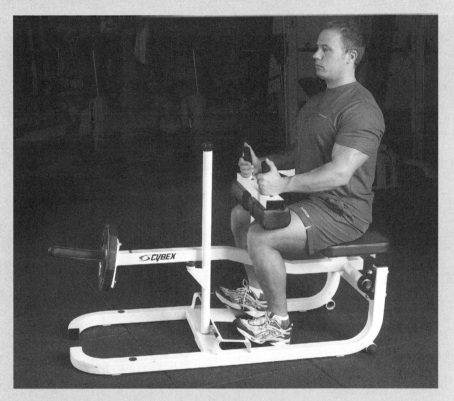

Starting position — heels on the ground.

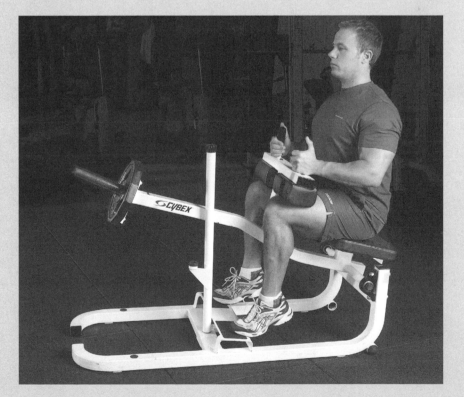

Raise the heels as high as possible.

Half-Seat Raise

BENEFITS: *Foot and ankle strength*

Equipment

- Half-round foam roller, block, or 2 x 4

How do I do this?

1. Stand upright with your feet slightly wider than shoulder width. Position the balls of your feet on a foam roller or block. This is your starting position.

2. Assume a half-seat position with your elbows bent and hands forward, as if holding the reins.

3. Once you have a balanced position, lower your heels while maintaining the half-seat.

4. Pause for 1 second at the bottom, then slowly return to your starting position.

5. Raise your heels as high as possible.

6. Pause for 1 second, then lower yourself to starting position.

7. Perform seven to ten repetitions.

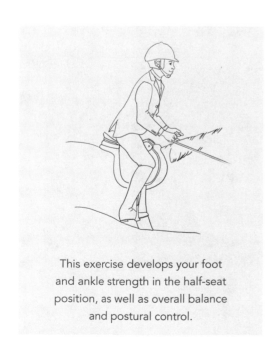

This exercise develops your foot and ankle strength in the half-seat position, as well as overall balance and postural control.

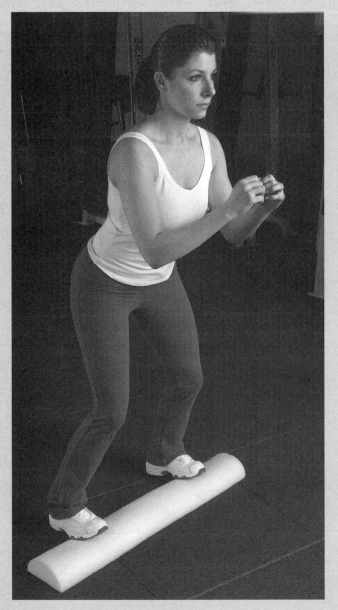

Maintain a balanced position with heels lowered.

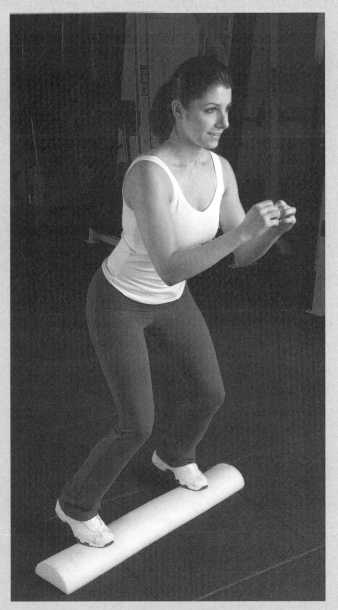

Maintain a balanced position with heels raised.

HINTS

- Keep your eyes focused ahead, as if looking to the next jump.
- Keep your back straight and your shoulders pulled back, as if mounted.

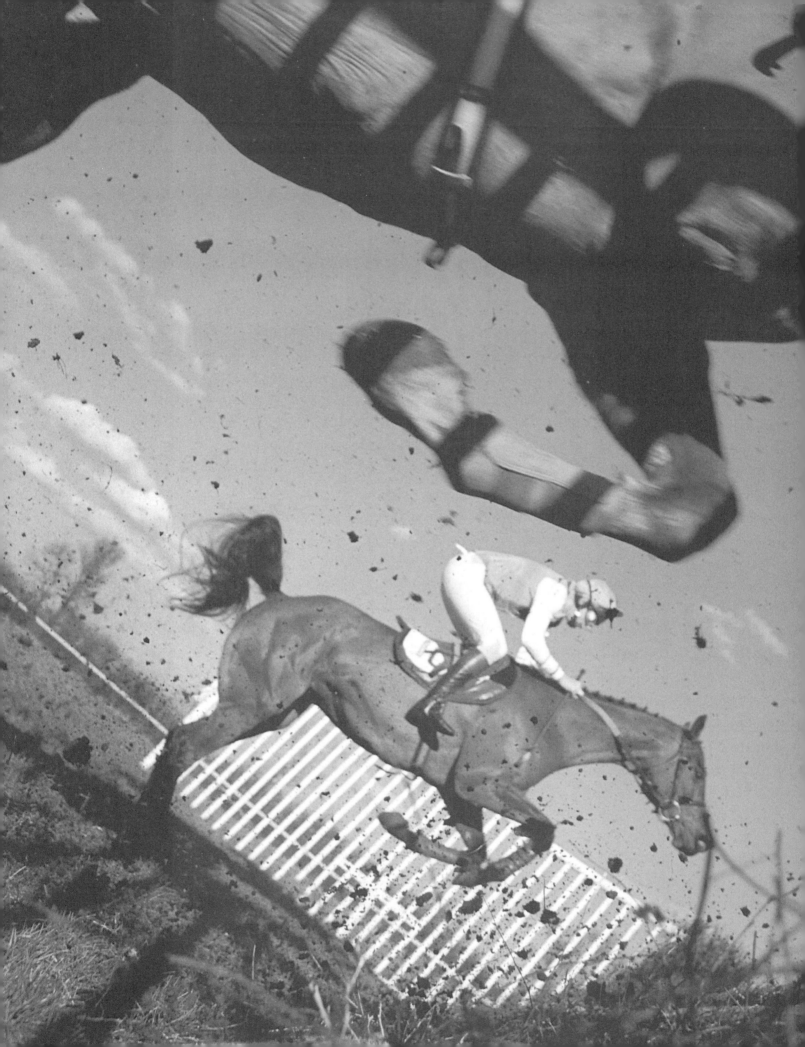

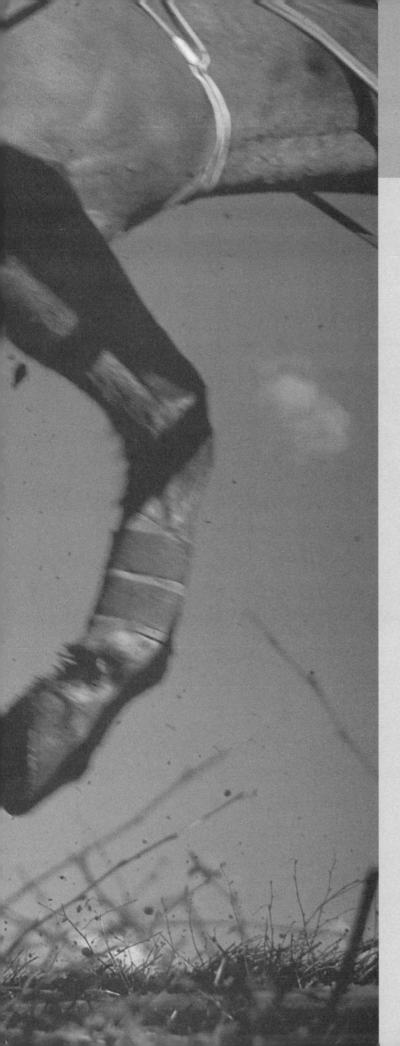

Chapter 4

PELVIC TILT

Strength and mobility in the pelvis, hips, and lower back are the keys to your connection with your horse. Your seat and legs are in constant communication with your horse, so stability and independence are important for effective aids.

Holding a galloping position, a full-seat position, a half-seat position, and jumping — both takeoff and landing, and especially landing on uneven, steep ground or in water — all depend on strong and flexible hips, pelvis, and lower back. Your lower back and pelvis also work as shock absorbers, especially in the sitting trot, when you need to appear as if you are not moving at all. Combined with your abdominal muscles, they improve your posture and balance and allow you to be independent with your aids for top performance.

All of these areas, especially your lower back, are prone to stress, fatigue, and injury. Incorporating strength and flexibility exercises into your everyday routine will make you a better rider and reduce the risk of future problems.

Hanging Knee Raise

BENEFIT: *Pelvic muscle strength*

Equipment

- Parallel dip bars

How do I do this?

1. On the hip-flexor station, support your body weight with your forearms, allowing your legs to hang straight down without touching the floor. If possible, position yourself away from the back support of the device.

2. Tilt your pelvis backward, as if trying to press the top of your sacrum up toward the ceiling.

3. Hold your pelvis in this position, then pull your legs up and in front of you, allowing your knees to bend as your legs are raised. Stop when your legs are directly in front of you, with your thighs parallel to the floor.

4. Lower your legs slowly, maintaining the pelvic tilt you established at the outset of the exercise.

5. Perform seven to ten repetitions.

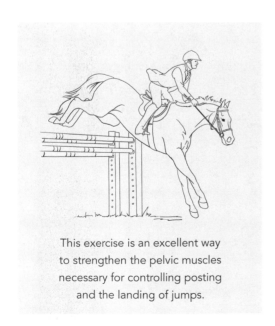

This exercise is an excellent way to strengthen the pelvic muscles necessary for controlling posting and the landing of jumps.

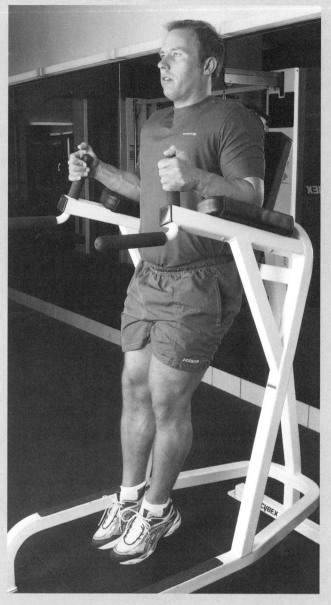

Starting position.

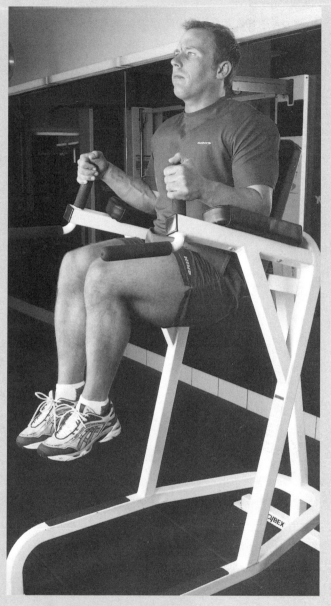

Knees up, thighs parallel to the floor.

HINTS

- Keep your body as still as possible throughout the movement.
- Slowly raise your legs forward, without swinging.
- Keep your back straight with your head and eyes up, as if mounted.

Incline Board Reverse Curl

BENEFITS: *Upper-body stability, abdominal strength*

Equipment

- Incline board

How do I do this?

1. Lie on your back with your head at the higher end of the incline board.

2. Reach overhead with your hands and grasp the handle above you. Lift up your legs with knees bent and press your lower back into the board.

3. While bending your knees, pull your legs up toward your chest.

4. As your knees reach your waist, roll your pelvis back, further elevating your knees toward your chin.

5. Hold this position for 1 second, then slowly return to the starting position.

6. Perform seven to ten repetitions.

HINTS

- Perform this exercise in a smooth and controlled manner.
- Be sure to keep your back flat and straight.

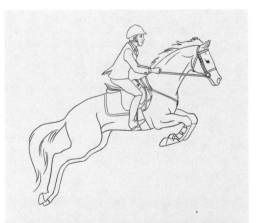

This exercise provides some upper-body stability and challenges you to engage the abdominal muscles that are critical to an effective pelvic position in the saddle.

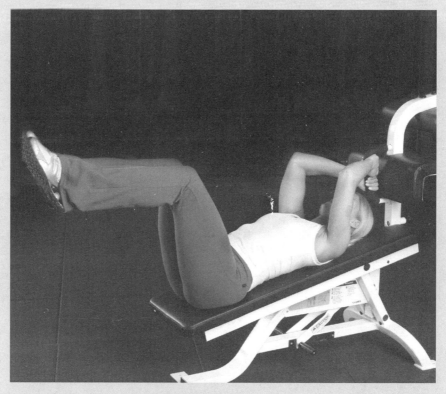

Starting position, knees bent and legs elevated.

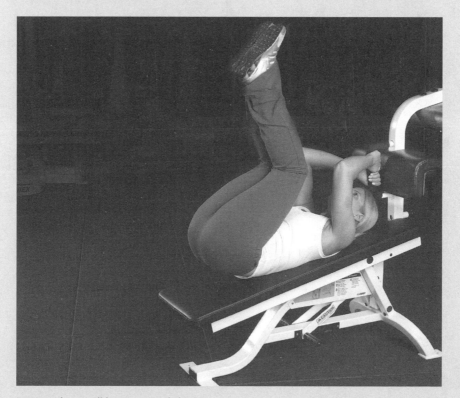

Legs to chest, roll knees toward chin.

Reciprocal Hanging Knee Raise

BENEFITS: *Pelvic control, abdominal strength*

Equipment

- Parallel dip bars

How do I do this?

1. On the hip-flexor station, support your body weight with your forearms, allowing your legs to hang straight down without touching the floor. Position yourself away from the back support of the device.

2. Holding your pelvis in a neutral position, pull one leg up and in front of you, allowing your knee to bend. Stop when your leg is directly in front of you, the thigh parallel to the floor. Your other leg should remain hanging straight down.

3. Lower your leg slowly, simultaneously raising the opposite leg at the same pace. Focus on keeping your pelvis in a fixed, neutral position.

4. Perform seven to ten repetitions.

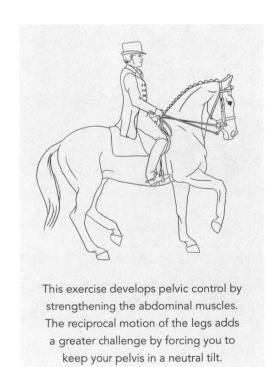

This exercise develops pelvic control by strengthening the abdominal muscles. The reciprocal motion of the legs adds a greater challenge by forcing you to keep your pelvis in a neutral tilt.

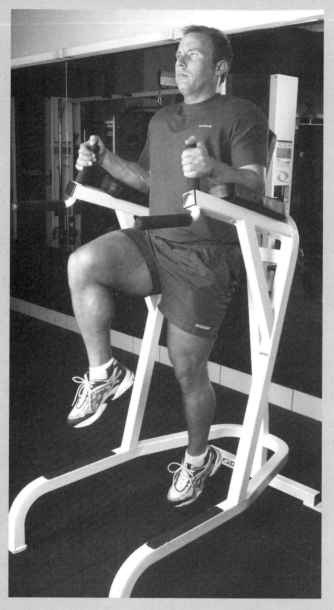

Raise right leg with a bent knee, thigh parallel to floor.

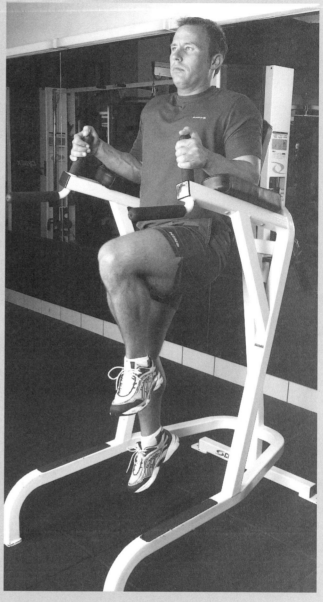

Left leg comes up as you slowly lower the right.

HINTS

- Keep your body as still as possible throughout the movement.
- Raise your legs slowly without swinging.
- Keep your back straight.

Counter Rotation

BENEFITS: Balance and stability

Equipment

- Tilt board
- Medicine ball

How do I do this?

1. Stand tall on a tilt board and establish your balance.

2. Hold your arms up and in front of you, as if holding the reins, or hold a medicine ball between your hands.

3. Rotate your trunk to the right. At the same time, rotate your pelvis to the left.

4. Return to center, then rotate the upper body and pelvis in the opposite directions.

5. Perform seven to ten repetitions.

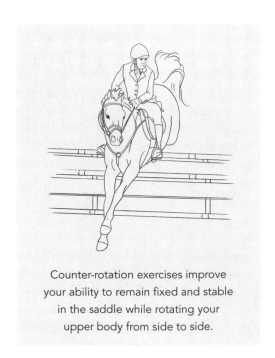

Counter-rotation exercises improve your ability to remain fixed and stable in the saddle while rotating your upper body from side to side.

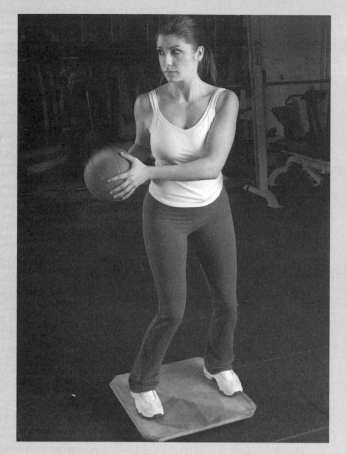

Rotate trunk to the right, pelvis to the left.

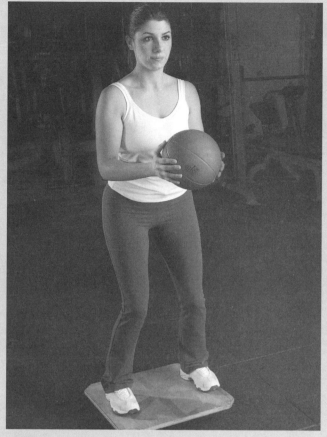

Center.

HINTS

- Stopping is as important as starting, so be sure to rotate to a point and then stop without going too far.
- Be sure your hands and arms are in the correct position — as if there is a straight line from your elbow to wrist to bit, with your hands held out, thumbs up, as if shaking someone else's hand.
- Holding a medicine ball will help you focus.

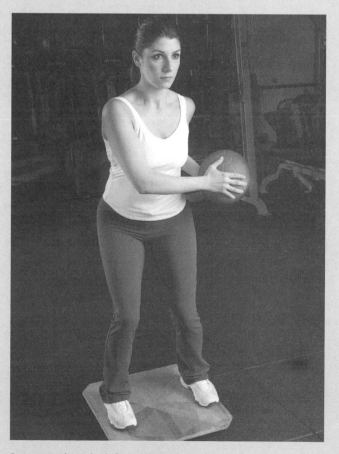

Rotate trunk to the left, pelvis to the right.

Trunk Curl with Rotation on a Physioball

BENEFITS: *Abdominal and trunk rotator strength*

Equipment

- Medium physioball

HINT

- Remember to keep your head in a neutral position with your eyes up and looking forward, as if mounted.

How do I do this?

1. Lie on your back with the physioball positioned under your lumbar region. Place your feet on the floor at approximately horse width.

2. Cross your arms over your chest. While keeping your head in a neutral position, curl your trunk forward and rotate to one side.

3. Slowly lower your trunk to the starting position.

4. Perform seven to ten repetitions. Repeat the set, rotating to the other side. Take a short pause between every second or third repetition.

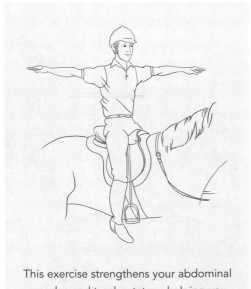

This exercise strengthens your abdominal muscles and trunk rotators, helping you establish and maintain a more balanced and stable position in the saddle.

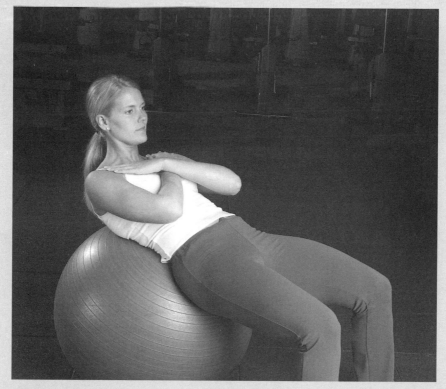

Starting position.

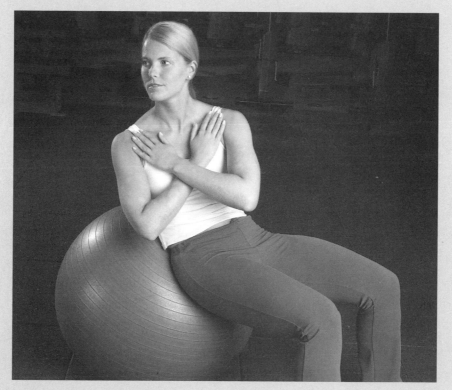

Trunk curl with a side rotation.

Trunk Curl with Alternate Knee Raise on a Physioball

BENEFITS: *Strength, balance*

Equipment

- Medium physioball

How do I do this?

1. Lie on your back with the physioball positioned under your lumbar region. Place your feet on the floor at approximately horse width.

2. Cross your arms over your chest and, keeping your head in a neutral position, curl your trunk forward and rotate to one side.

3. Simultaneously, raise the leg on the side to which you are rotating.

4. As you lower your trunk to the starting position, return your leg to the floor.

5. Repeat on the opposite side.

6. Perform seven to ten repetitions on each side.

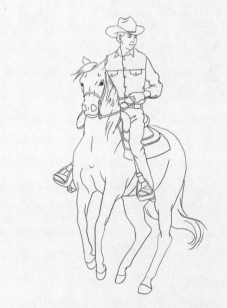

This core strengthening exercise is enhanced by the unstable physioball. The added torso stability and pelvic control will translate into an improved posting posture and a greater ability to absorb forces through your body when landing after jumps.

HINTS

- Be sure to keep your head in a neutral position. Think about your mounted posture and keeping your eyes looking ahead.
- If you feel too unstable, start with a small range of motion, then gradually increase your range.

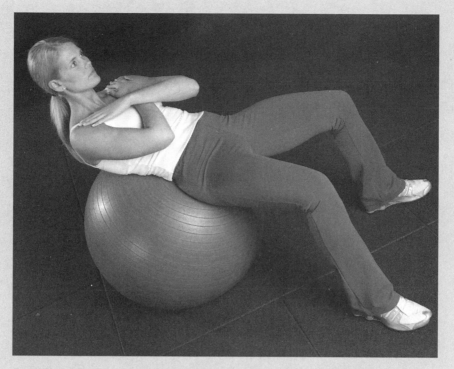

Starting position.

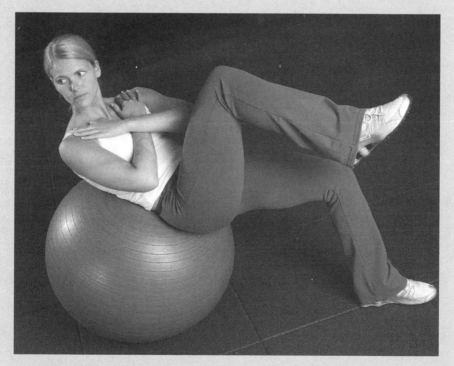

Trunk curl with knee raise.

Alternate Leg Lowering on an Incline Board

BENEFITS: *Strengthens hip and pelvic muscles*

Equipment

- Incline board

HINT

- Keep your pelvis in a neutral tilt during this exercise, being sure to keep it still while lowering the leg.

How do I do this?

1. Lie on your back with your head at the higher end of the incline board.

2. Reach overhead with your hands and grasp the handle above you. Press your lower back into the board.

3. While bending your knees, pull up your legs toward your chest.

4. From the legs-up position, extend and lower one leg until it is just above the floor; keep the other leg up.

5. Bring the extended leg back to the up position, then extend and lower the other leg.

6. Perform seven to ten repetitions.

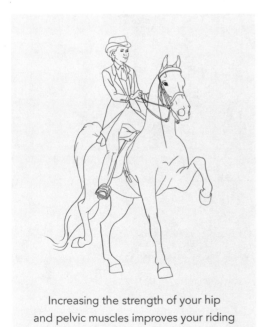

Increasing the strength of your hip and pelvic muscles improves your riding position and posting.

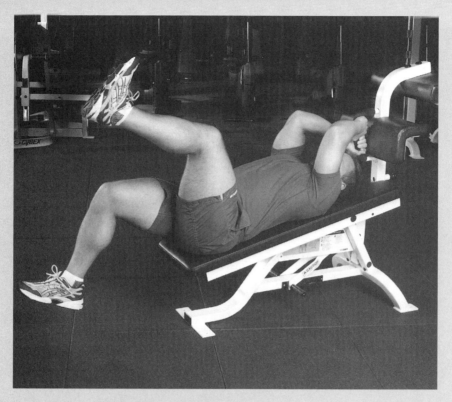

Lower one leg while keeping the other elevated.

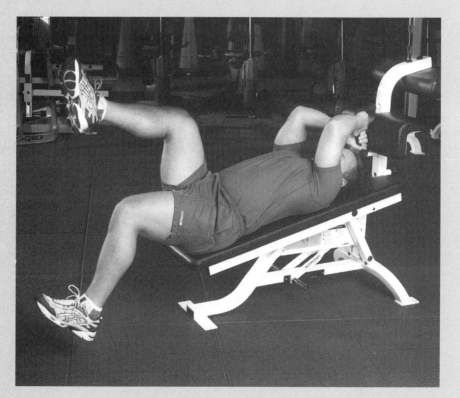

Alternate.

Dynamic Pelvic Control

BENEFIT: *Pelvic stability*

Equipment

- Mat
- Partner

HINT

- Keep your head on the floor and your back flat, and focus on preventing motion around your hips and pelvis.

Note: This is a difficult exercise and potentially stressful to the lumbar spine. Use caution when doing it.

How do I do this?

1. Lie on your back on the mat with a partner standing with one foot on either side of your head, facing your legs. Bring up your legs so that they are vertical and your partner can grab your feet. Your knees should be slightly bent.

2. Widen your legs to approximately shoulder width and place your arms on the floor by your sides.

3. Have your partner push your legs toward the floor in a short, quick thrust. Stabilize your pelvis and legs against the thrust. Bring your legs to a smooth stop before touching the floor.

4. Return to starting position, then repeat two or three times.

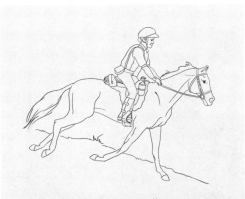

This exercise is an excellent way to establish stability around the pelvis, improving your tolerance for sudden stresses while in the saddle. It requires the assistance of a training partner.

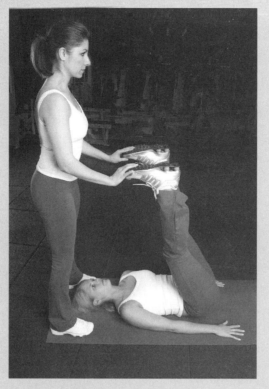

Starting position.

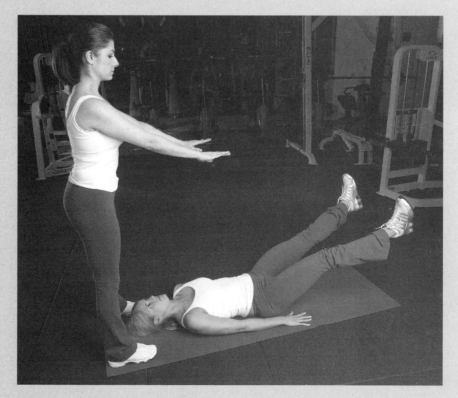

Maintain control through the torso while responding to thrusts.

Pelvic Clock

BENEFIT: *Pelvic control*

Equipment

• Mat

How do I do this?

1. Lie on your back on the floor. Bend your knees, placing your feet flat on the floor, with your heels about 12 inches from your buttocks.

2. Imagine a clock face under your pelvis, with the 12 toward your head, the 6 toward your feet, and the 3 and 9 at either side.

3. Moving clockwise, slowly rotate your pelvis, tilting it so that it touches each number on the clock.

4. Repeat in a counterclockwise direction.

5. Repeat again, touching random numbers around the clock, two or three times at each number. Rest and repeat again.

This basic pelvic exercise helps to establish movement control, which is an essential building block for all other pelvic exercises.

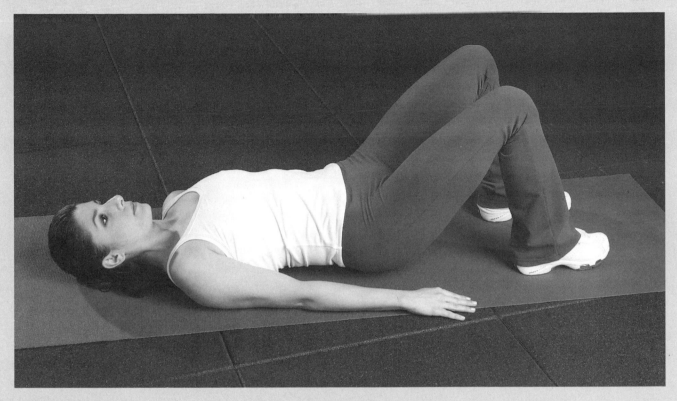

Starting position.

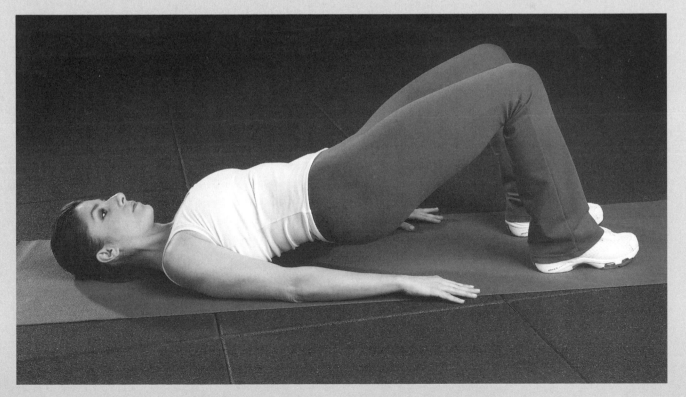

Tilt the pelvis to each position on the clock.

Seated Physioball Hula

BENEFIT: *Lateral torso stability*

Equipment

- Large physioball

How do I do this?

1. Sit on the center of a large physioball with your feet shoulder-width apart.

2. Raise your arms in an oval shape above your head.

3. Push your pelvis to one side, so that the ball rolls slightly in the opposite direction.

4. Use your pelvic muscles to return to the center, then push to the opposite side.

5. Perform seven to ten repetitions.

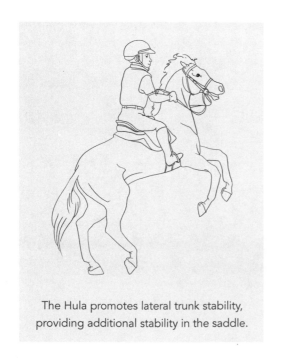

The Hula promotes lateral trunk stability, providing additional stability in the saddle.

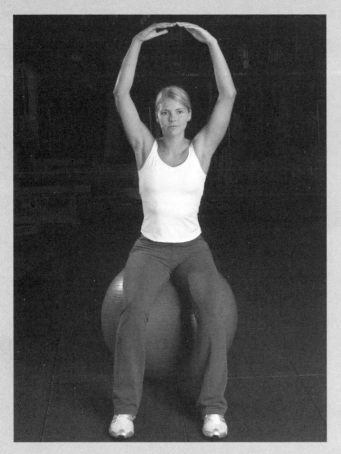

Starting position.

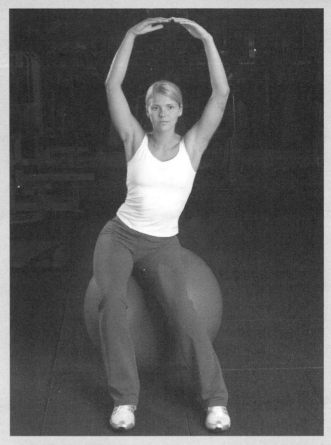

Push pelvis to the right.

HINTS

- Keep your body upright and aligned and your back flat.
- If necessary, place your hands on the ball in order to control lateral motion.

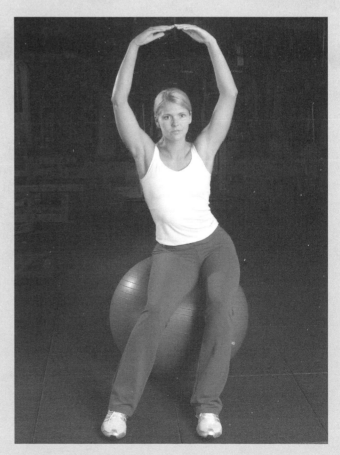

Shift to the left.

Seated Physioball Back and Forth

BENEFITS: *Strength and pelvic rhythm*

Equipment

- Large physioball

How do I do this?

1. Sit on the center of a large physioball with your legs in front of you, slightly narrower than hip width, and your feet on the floor 24 inches in front of the ball.

2. Press your feet into the floor and push the ball backward while inclining your trunk slightly forward.

3. Use your pelvic muscles to pull the ball forward to the starting position, then continue to use these muscles to push the ball slightly forward.

4. Perform seven to ten repetitions.

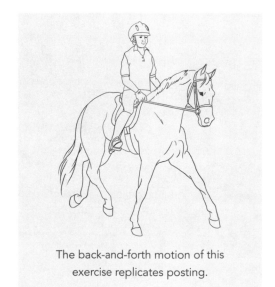

The back-and-forth motion of this exercise replicates posting.

CHALLENGE

Increase the difficulty of this exercise by crossing your arms in front of your chest. This prevents you from using your arms for balance, thus increasing their independence — a necessity for good riding!

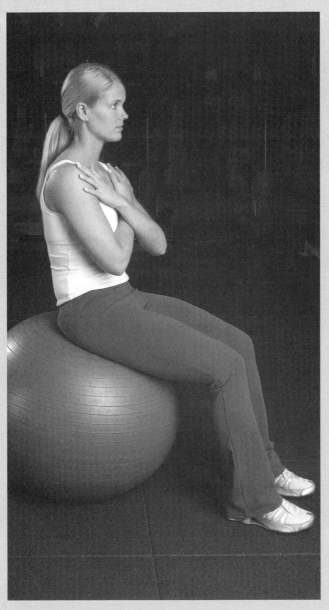

Push the ball back with a slight trunk incline.

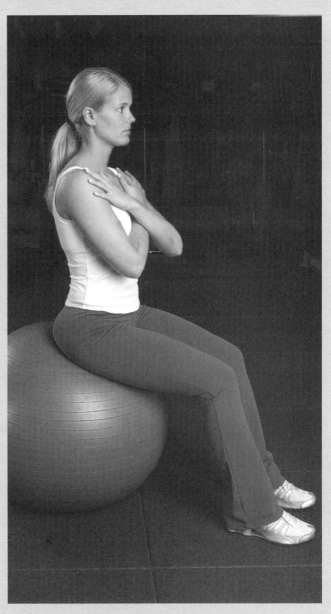

Return to starting position by pulling the ball forward.

HINT

- Keep your trunk upright and aligned; do not round your spine.

Physioball Scale

BENEFITS: *Abdominal- and back-muscle strength, upper-body stability*

Equipment

- Large physioball

How do I do this?

1. Sit on the center of a large physioball with your legs in front of you, slightly narrower than hip width, and your feet on the floor 24 inches in front of the ball.

2. Raise your arms in an oval shape above your head.

3. Pull the ball toward your heels and tilt your trunk backward as far as you can while maintaining balance on the ball.

4. Push the ball backward, allowing your trunk to incline forward.

5. Return to starting position, then perform seven to ten repetitions.

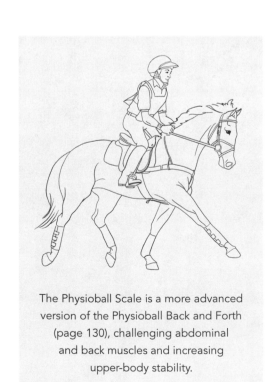

The Physioball Scale is a more advanced version of the Physioball Back and Forth (page 130), challenging abdominal and back muscles and increasing upper-body stability.

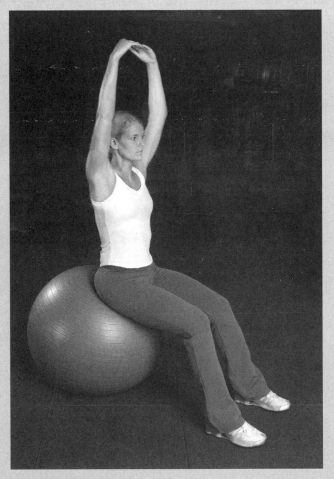

Starting position.

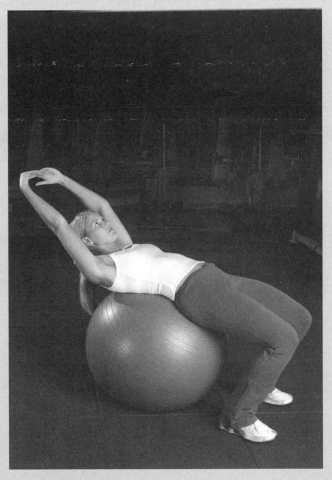

Pull ball forward while tilting trunk back.

HINT

- Keep the spine straight and the shoulders back, as if mounted.

Trunk Extension with Rotation on Physioball

BENEFIT: *Lower-back strength*

Equipment

- Large physioball

HINTS

- Try to maintain a smooth motion during this exercise.
- Be sure to extend your body before you rotate the trunk.

How do I do this?

1. Lie facedown on a large physioball positioned beneath your abdomen.

2. Spread your legs to shoulder width, keeping the balls of your feet on the floor.

3. Place your hands on either side of your head.

4. To start, allow your trunk to bend forward, following the curve of the ball.

5. Extend your trunk up and off the ball, until your back is straight and slightly above horizontal. As you approach the extended position, rotate your trunk slightly to one side.

6. Return to the starting position, then repeat on the other side.

7. Perform seven to ten repetitions on each side.

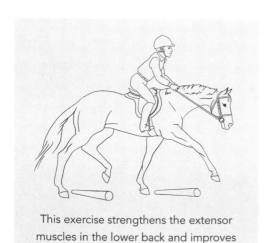

This exercise strengthens the extensor muscles in the lower back and improves riding posture.

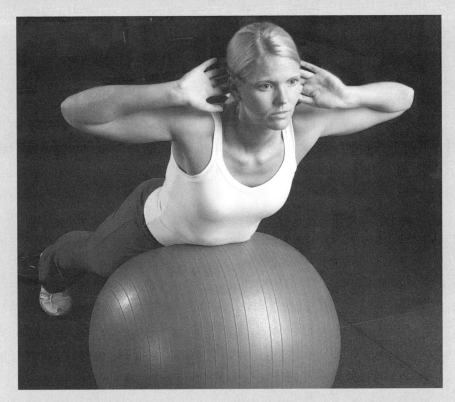

Trunk angled above the physioball.

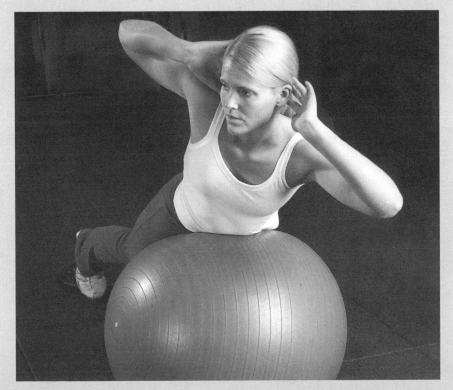

Trunk rotation.

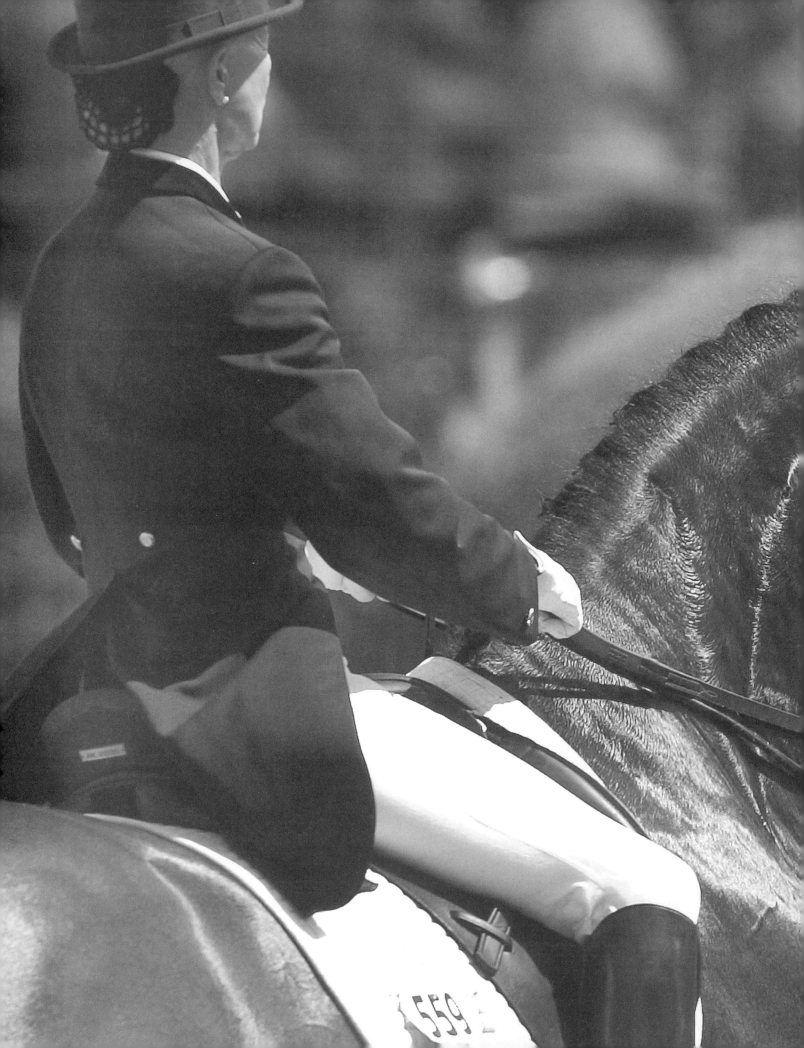

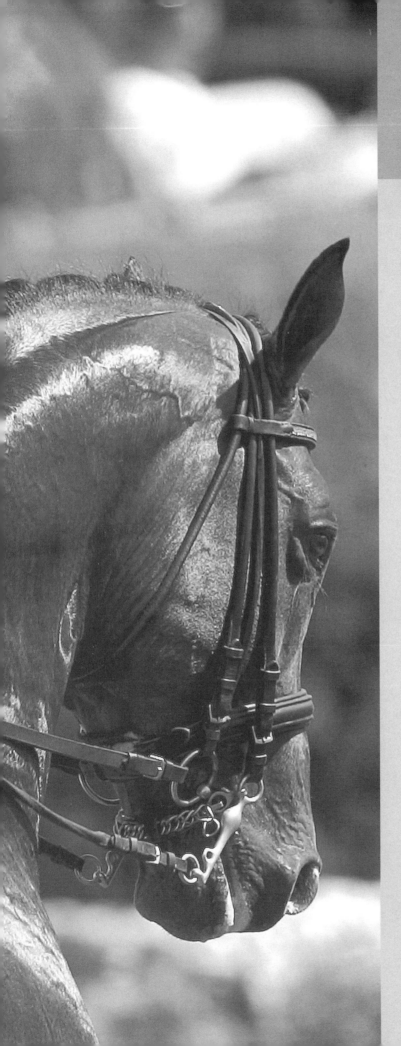

Chapter 5

POSTURE

Your posture directly affects your communication with your horse by influencing your balance. A rider with a long torso and short legs struggles with posture far more than a rider with long legs and a short torso. All of us struggle to some extent; keeping our bodies straight — back flat, shoulders open, head up, and eyes looking where we want to go — is crucial to proper communication with our horses and it allows us to breathe and relax, especially in a competitive situation.

Many of these exercises use a physioball or medicine ball to replicate the unsteady nature of riding a horse — a form of multitasking that will improve your posture and your riding. Making good posture the norm will help prevent upper-back, neck, and shoulder injuries, and allow clear breathing, relaxation, and concentration.

Shoulder Rotation with Physioball

BENEFITS: *Shoulder coordination and stability*

Equipment

- Large physioball

CHALLENGE

Try this exercise in a downward-facing, push-up position.

How do I do this?

1. Stand approximately 3 feet in front of a wall.

2. While grasping a physioball, stretch your arms in front of you just below shoulder height.

3. Lean forward so that the ball is pressed into the wall. Your body weight should lean into the ball.

4. Using only the shoulder muscles, rotate the ball in a counterclockwise direction for several repetitions.

5. Repeat the motion in the opposite direction.

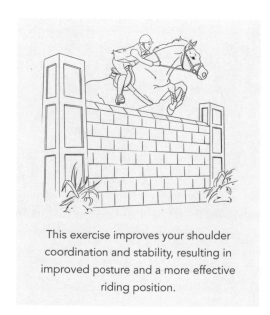

This exercise improves your shoulder coordination and stability, resulting in improved posture and a more effective riding position.

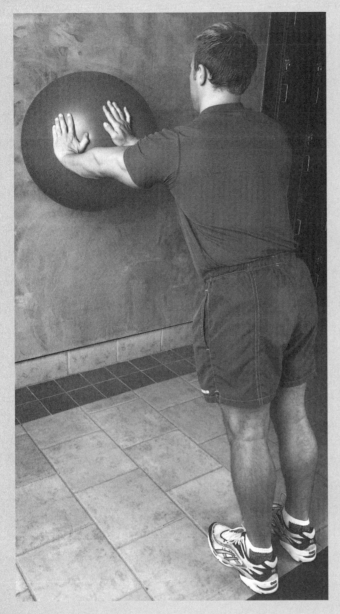

Starting position.

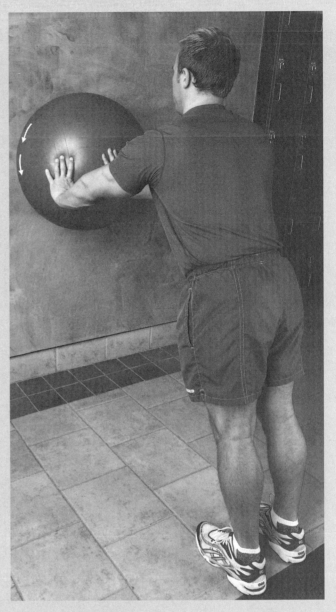

Rotate using the shoulder muscles.

HINTS

- Keep your elbows straight.
- Keep your trunk and hips stable as you rotate the ball.

Seated Dumbbell Front Raise on Physioball

BENEFIT: *Posture stabilization*

Equipment

- Large physioball
- Dumbbells

How do I do this?

1. Sit up straight on a physioball with your feet at approximately shoulder width. Keep your pelvis straight and your back upright.

2. Hold the dumbbells at your sides.

3. Elevate your arms until they are level with your shoulders and directly in front of you.

4. Pause for 1 second, then lower to the starting position.

5. Perform seven to ten repetitions.

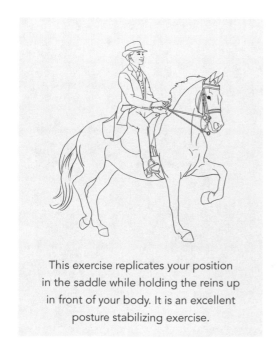

This exercise replicates your position in the saddle while holding the reins up in front of your body. It is an excellent posture stabilizing exercise.

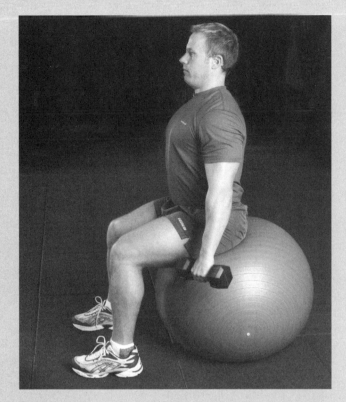

Starting position.

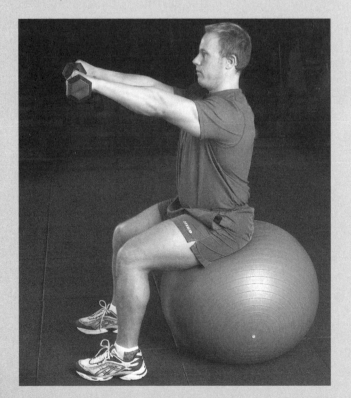

Elevate arms in front.

Seated Row on Physioball

BENEFITS: *Posture, shoulder strength*

Equipment

- Large physioball
- Adjustable pulley system with a handle or elastic tubing, anchored in the middle so it creates two strands

How do I do this?

1. Sit on the physioball, facing the pulley or tubing anchor point. Set the pulley or anchor the tubing level to your shoulders. Your feet should be positioned in front of you and 12 to 24 inches apart.

2. Grasp the pulley handle or the tubing ends with one hand and sit upright, so that the cable or tube is taut. Your arm should be outstretched in front of you.

3. Keeping your back straight and your head up, pull the handle toward you, leading with your elbow, so that your hand comes in close to your torso.

4. Pause for 1 second, then slowly return the handle to the starting position.

5. Perform seven to ten repetitions with each arm.

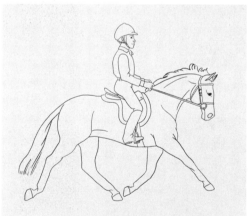

The Seated Row develops your posterior shoulder strength, improving your control of the reins and thus your feel for the horse's mouth. Because the exercise is done in a seated position, greater emphasis is placed on your upper-body position and posture control, translating to better balance when mounted. The ball adds an element of instability, forcing you to control your balance and posture.

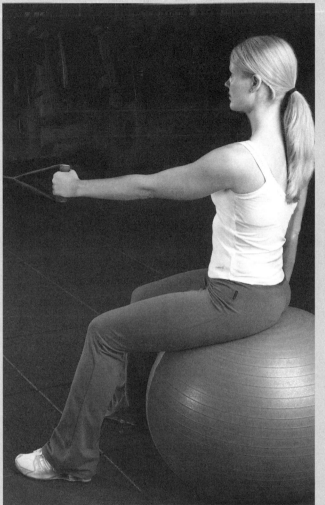

Starting position.

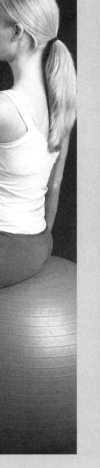

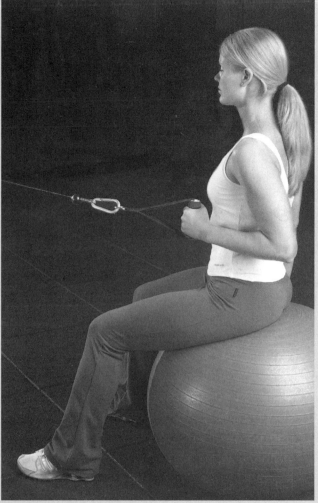

Pull through leading with the elbow.

HINTS

- Focus on remaining balanced and keeping an erect posture.
- Be sure to keep your pelvis and spine upright.
- Be sure to pull back your shoulders before moving your arms.
- Keep the ball as still as possible, using your trunk and hips to maintain your position.

Timed Wall Squat with Trunk Rotation

BENEFITS: Endurance, strength, posture

Equipment

- Two medicine balls weighing between 2 and 6 pounds
- Large physioball

This complex exercise challenges your endurance, saddle position, and posture, all at the same time. It is excellent for helping you contend with the myriad challenges experienced while executing a course.

How do I do this?

1. Stand with your back approximately 3 feet from a wall.

2. Place one medicine ball between your legs, just above your knees, and squeeze your legs to hold the ball.

3. Place the physioball behind your pelvis, then sit back into the ball, pressing it against the wall. Your body should assume a seated position, with your back vertical, your thighs parallel to the floor, and your knees bent at a 90-degree angle.

4. Continue to squeeze your legs together to keep the medicine ball fixed between your legs.

5. Hold the second medicine ball in your hands and raise your arms in front of you, keeping your elbows straight.

6. Without moving your arms, rotate your trunk as far as possible to one side without losing balance. The physioball will move slightly in the opposite direction. Do not allow it to fall to the floor.

7. Move up and down slightly, as if creating a modified posting motion.

8. While pulsing up and down, rotate your trunk completely to the opposite side, keeping your arms extended in front of you and the ball fixed between your legs.

9. Rotate back and forth for 30 seconds.

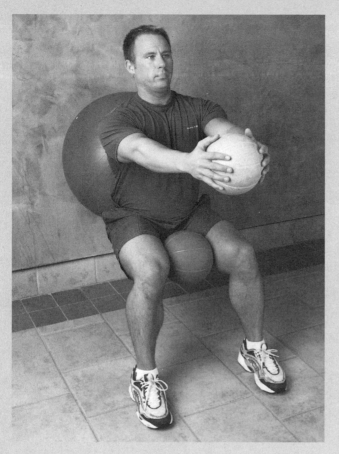

Starting position.

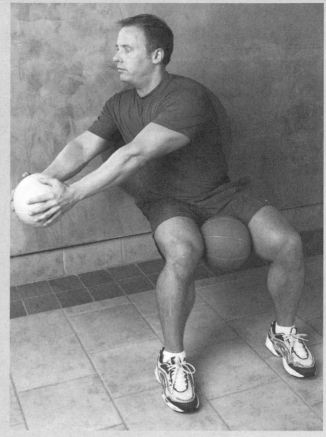

Trunk rotation to the right.

HINTS

- Look straight ahead, as if mounted.
- Keep your back straight and your shoulders square.
- Feel your body weight through your insteps. If you sense it toward your toes, you'll need to move your feet farther from the wall. If your weight is over your heels, bring your feet closer to the wall.

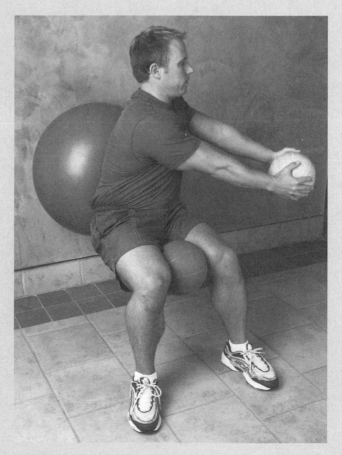

Rotate trunk to the left.

Russian Twist with Medicine Ball

BENEFITS: *Upper-body stabilization and control*

Equipment

- Mat
- 2- to 4-pound medicine ball

CHALLENGE

Slide your feet closer to your body to increase the challenge.

The Russian Twist is an excellent trunk-stabilizing movement that promotes upper-body control and postural integrity. Forces that push you back into the saddle will be handled efficiently and effectively, thus giving you better stability when mounted.

How do I do this?

1. Sit on the mat with your knees bent and your feet flat. Your heels should be approximately 24 inches from your buttocks. Slide your feet farther from you if necessary to make it easier to maintain this position.

2. Place a medicine ball on the floor next to your left hip. Keeping your spine straight, lean back slightly until you feel your abdominal muscles contract to keep you from falling back. If your lower back begins to strain, sit more upright.

3. Rotate your trunk toward the medicine ball and grasp it.

4. Using only your trunk, rotate to the right side, touching the medicine ball to the floor next to your right hip.

5. Perform seven to ten repetitions in both directions.

HINTS

- Be sure to keep your spine elongated and your pelvis upright.
- If you find yourself falling back, move your feet farther forward.

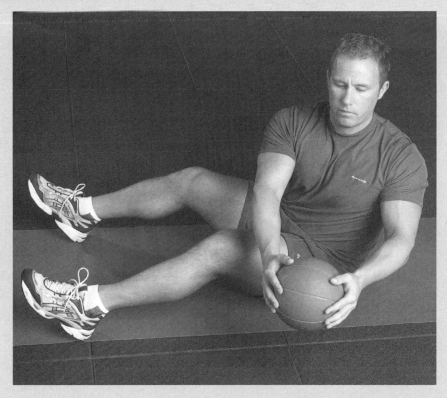

Grasp the ball with a trunk rotation.

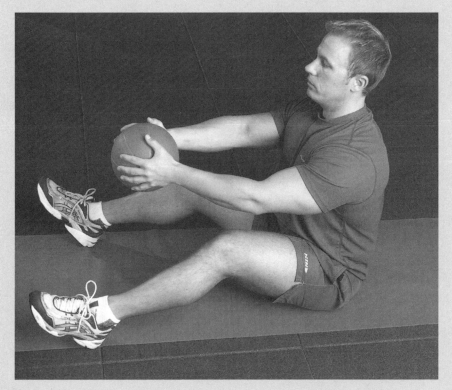

Holding the ball, rotate to the other side.

Side Plank

BENEFIT: Posture

Equipment

- Mat

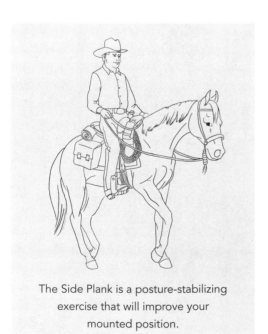

The Side Plank is a posture-stabilizing exercise that will improve your mounted position.

How do I do this?

1. Lie on your side on the mat, with your body aligned so that your top arm and leg form a straight line.

2. Position your bottom forearm perpendicular to the line of your body, hand pointing forward, and prop yourself up so that your arm forms a right angle to your body. Your trunk should be angled up away from the floor while your legs and hips remain in contact with it.

3. Keeping your trunk firm and your arm rigid, lift your hips off the floor until your body forms a straight line from shoulders to ankles.

4. Hold this position for 1 second, then lower your hips to the floor.

5. Perform seven to ten repetitions, then repeat on the other side.

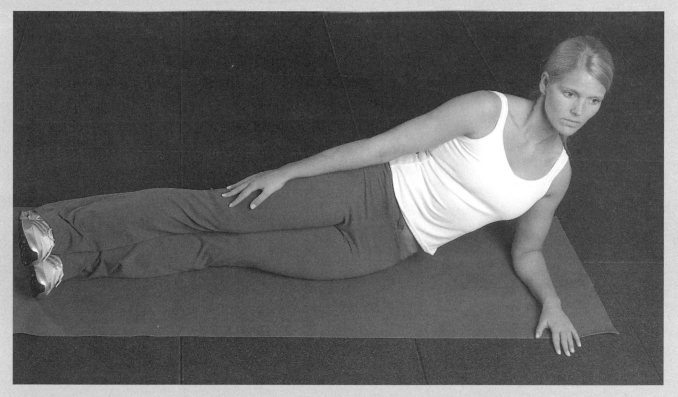

Starting position.

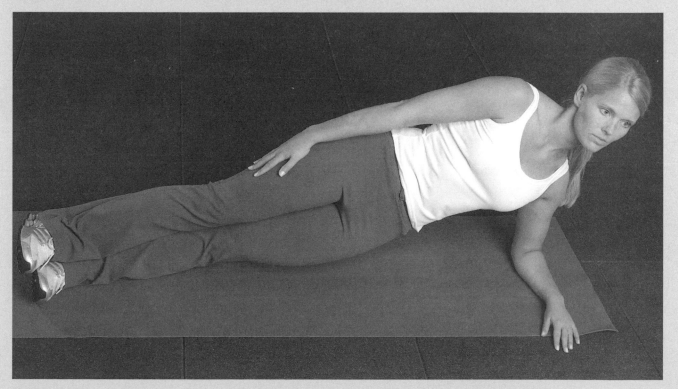

Lift hips off the floor.

Side Plank with DynaDisc

BENEFITS: Posture and balance

Equipment

- Mat
- DynaDisc

HINTS

- Keep your supporting shoulder as still as possible.
- Your movements should be smooth and controlled.

This exercise adds the challenge of an unstable surface under your supporting arm to the simple Side Plank exercise (page 148).

How do I do this?

1. Lie on your side on the mat, with your body aligned so that your top arm and leg form a straight line.

2. Place a DynaDisc beneath your bottom arm and position that forearm perpendicular to the line of your body, hand pointing forward, and prop yourself up so that your arm forms a right angle to your body. Your trunk should be angled up away from the floor while your legs and hips remain in contact with it.

3. Keeping your trunk firm and your arm rigid, lift your hips off the floor until your body forms a straight line from shoulders to ankles.

4. Hold this position for 1 second, then lower your hips to the floor.

5. Perform seven to ten repetitions, then repeat on the other side.

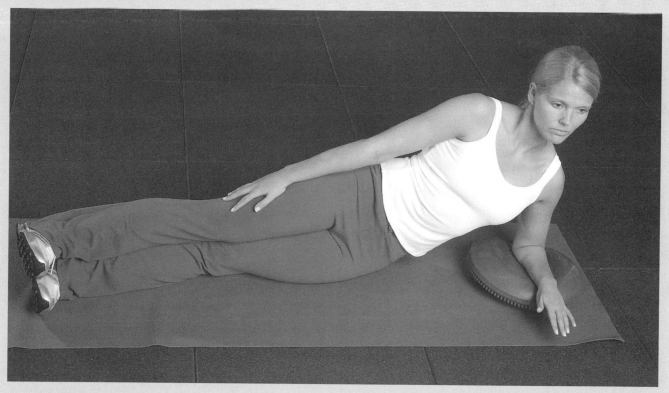

Starting position.

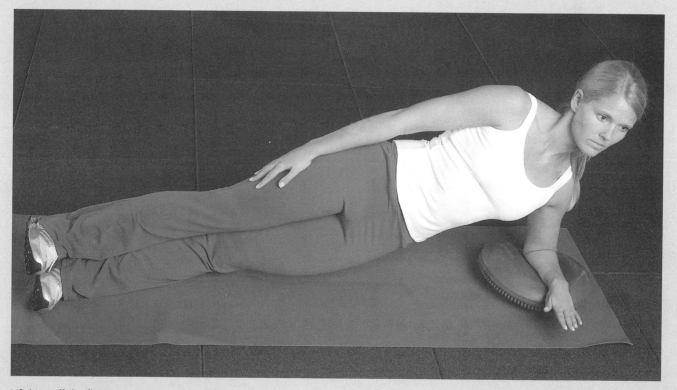

Lift hips off the floor.

Side Bending on a Half-Round

BENEFITS: *Strengthens trunk stabilizers*

Equipment

- Half-round foam roller
- Dumbbell

CHALLENGE

- Bring your feet closer together for an increased challenge.
- Stand on the flat side of the foam roller for a less stable position.

How do I do this?

1. Stand on the curved side of a half-round foam roller with your feet just less than shoulder-width apart.

2. Grasp a dumbbell in one hand and place your other hand at your side.

3. Lean to the side of the dumbbell, tilting sideways as far as you can without losing your balance.

4. Return to standing position.

5. Perform seven to ten repetitions, then repeat on the other side.

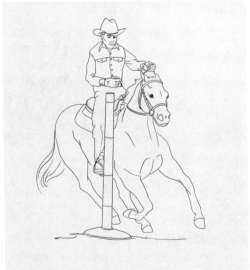

Side Bending on a Half-Round helps to strengthen the trunk stabilizers for a taller, more efficient position in the saddle.

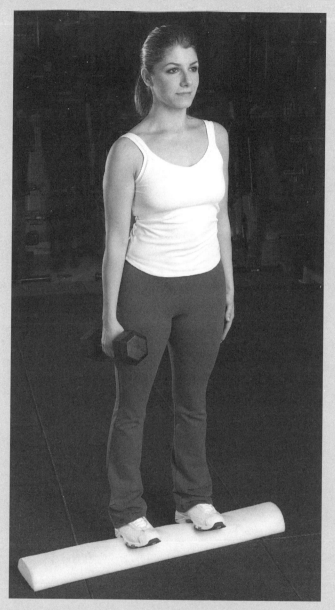

Starting position.

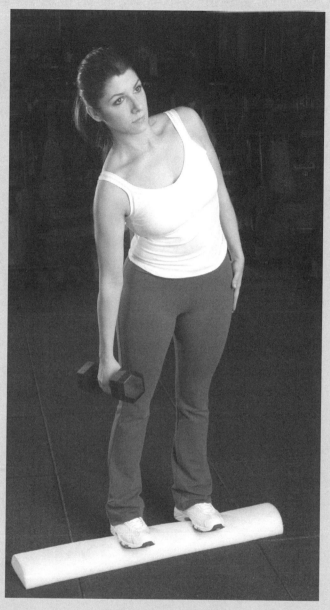

Maintain your balance with the bend.

HINT

- Keep your spine as straight and still as possible.

Trunk Extension

BENEFITS: *Posture, upper-body strength*

Equipment

- Mat

How do I do this?

1. Lie on your stomach on the mat with your arms positioned along your sides. Check to see that your shoulders are touching the mat. Align your head with your spine by placing your forehead on the mat.

2. Keeping your head aligned with your spine, extend and lift your trunk 2 to 3 inches off the floor.

3. Pause for a moment at the top, then return to the floor.

4. Perform seven to ten repetitions.

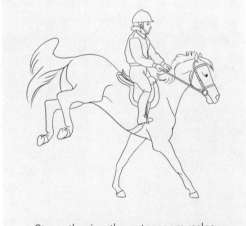

Strengthening the extensor muscles along the spine helps you maintain better posture, and will give you the ability to manage more effectively the forces pulling you forward on the horse.

HINT

- Avoid leading with your head or tilting your head too far backward.

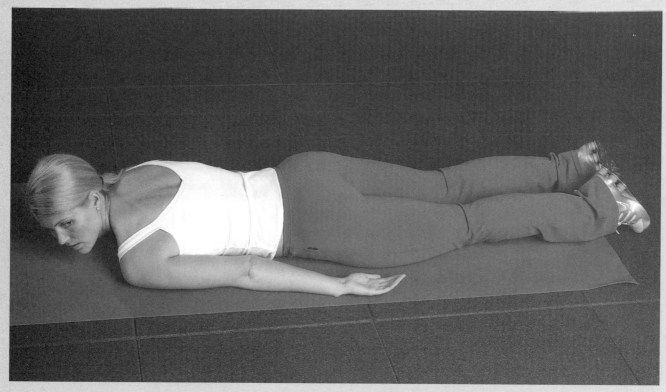

Shoulders are flat and arms positioned at sides.

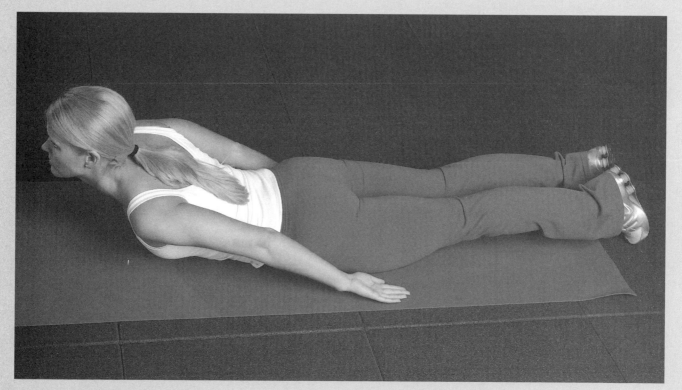

Align your head and lift your trunk.

Trunk Extension with Rotation

BENEFITS: *Upper-body strength and stability*

Equipment

- Mat

How do I do this?

1. Lie on your stomach on the mat with your arms positioned along your sides.

2. Keeping your head aligned with your spine, extend and lift your trunk 2 to 3 inches off the floor. As you approach the highest point, rotate your trunk slightly in one direction.

3. Pause for a moment at the top, then return to the floor.

4. Repeat, rotating in the opposite direction.

5. Perform seven to ten repetitions.

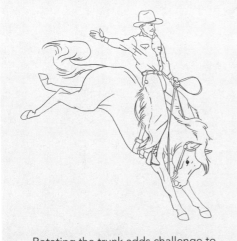

Rotating the trunk adds challenge to the simpler Trunk Extension exercise (page 154). This added dimension increases trunk stability and stress tolerance while riding.

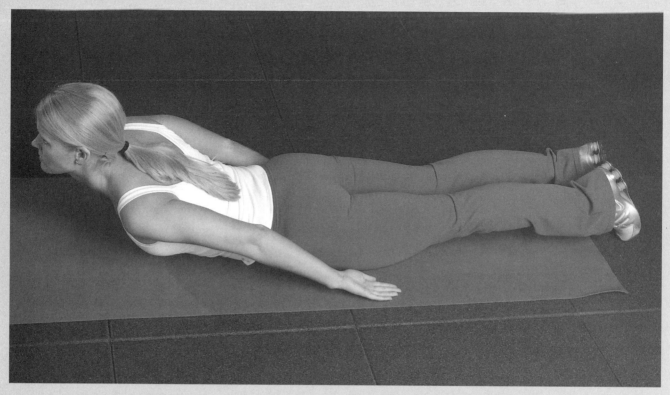

Lift trunk off floor.

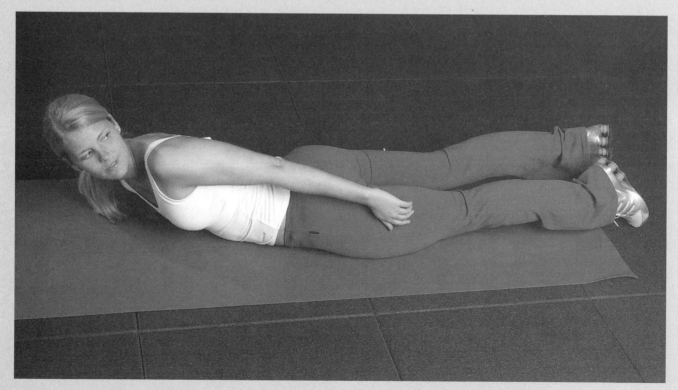

Rotate in one direction.

Medicine Ball Swing

BENEFIT: *Upper-body stability*

Equipment

- Medicine ball

How do I do this?

1. Stand with your feet approximately horse-width apart. Bend your knees into a high squat position.

2. Grasp the handles of the medicine ball and with your arms straight, reach down and back until the ball is between your feet.

3. Using the trunk to initiate motion, swing the medicine ball forward and up until it is directly over your head, extending your legs straight as you lift. Be very deliberate in stopping the ball overhead; the momentum of the ball should not cause your trunk to extend.

4. Swing the ball back downward between your feet, stopping deliberately at the bottom of the arc.

5. Perform seven to ten repetitions.

The Medicine Ball Swing mimics the horse's acceleration and deceleration — forward and backward forces that act on your upper body when riding. This leads to substantial increases in body control while posting, starting and stopping, and landing after jumps.

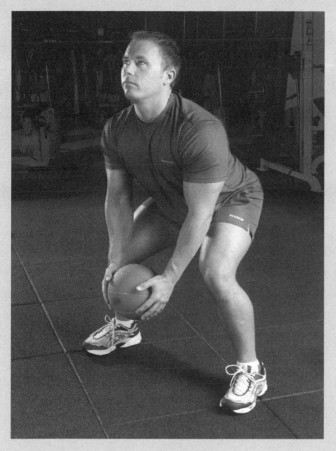

Starting position.

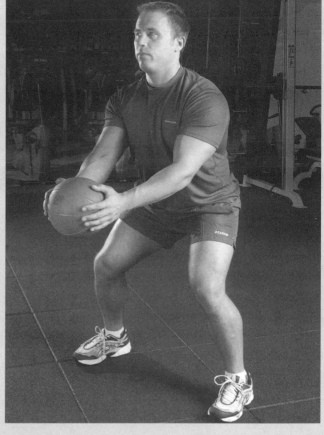

Swing forward and up.

HINTS

- Keep your shoulders and back straight.
- Always keep your weight stable and centered over your feet.

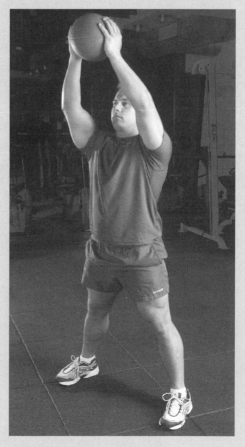

Stop overhead.

Combo Squat with Low-to-High Pull

BENEFITS: Upper- and lower-body strength and coordination, posture

Equipment

- Pulley system set near the floor or elastic tubing anchored near the floor

How do I do this?

1. Grab the pulley or tube handle, then step back so that you are standing approximately 3 feet from the pulley or tubing anchor point.

2. Lower your body toward the floor in the squat, keeping your weight centered over your feet. As you descend, your arms will be pulled slightly forward by the weight or elastic tubing; be sure to maintain your weight over the center of your feet.

3. Once in a comfortably lowered position, push down into the floor with your legs to return to a standing position.

4. As you approach the standing position, pull the handles toward your chin, leading with your elbows. When fully erect, your hands should be under your chin with your elbows pulled behind you.

5. Slowly extend your arms toward the pulley and lower yourself back into the squat position.

6. Perform seven to ten repetitions.

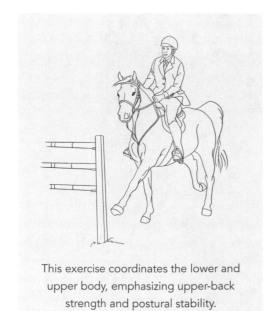

This exercise coordinates the lower and upper body, emphasizing upper-back strength and postural stability.

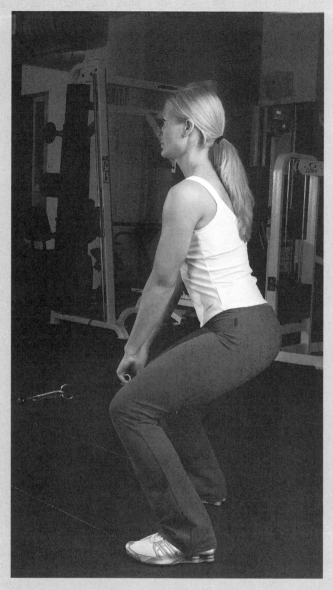

Lower to a squat (step 2).

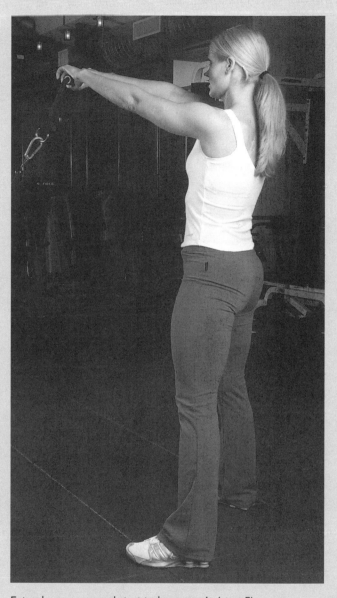

Extend your arms and start to lower again (step 5).

HINTS

- Look straight ahead with your eyes focused in front of you, as if riding.
- Keep your back and shoulders straight and square; double-check your posture before each phase of the exercise.

Quadruped Trunk Extension

BENEFIT: *Balance*

Equipment

- Mat

How do I do this?

1. Begin on your hands and knees, establishing a well-balanced and stable position.

2. Remove one hand from the floor, then rotate your trunk to the same side as far as possible without losing your balance.

3. Hold that position for 1 second, then return to the starting position.

4. Repeat on the opposite side.

5. Perform seven to ten repetitions on both sides.

HINTS
• Always stop rotating at the onset of any discomfort. • Keep your head aligned with your spine. • Use your trunk to move, and avoid swinging your arm.

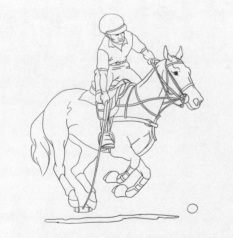

Performed on all fours, the Quadruped Trunk Extension adds a balance challenge to the simpler Trunk Extension exercise (page 154).

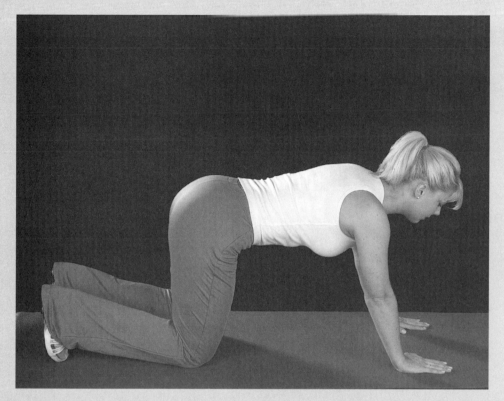

Starting position — all fours.

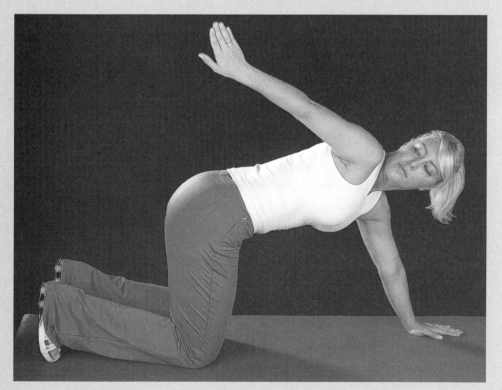

Extend arm and rotate trunk.

Prone Trunk Extension on Physioball with Shoulder Extension

BENEFITS: *Stability, balance*

Equipment

- Three-foot length of elastic band (not tubing)
- Large physioball

CHALLENGE

Bring your feet closer together.

How do I do this?

1. Place one end of the elastic band under the physioball.

2. Lie facedown with the physioball positioned at your midsection. Your legs should be stretched out behind you, with your feet shoulder-width apart, toes touching the floor.

3. Grab the loose end of the elastic band with one hand and keep the other hand on the ball.

4. Extend your back so that your body forms a straight line, then pull the band up and forward so that your arm extends straight, following the line of your body.

5. Return to the starting position, then perform seven to ten repetitions before doing the exercise on the other side.

HINTS

- Keep your head in line with your body.
- Try to keep the ball still. You may use your free hand to help stabilize the ball.

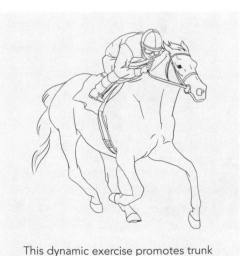

This dynamic exercise promotes trunk stability, balance, and shoulder stability.

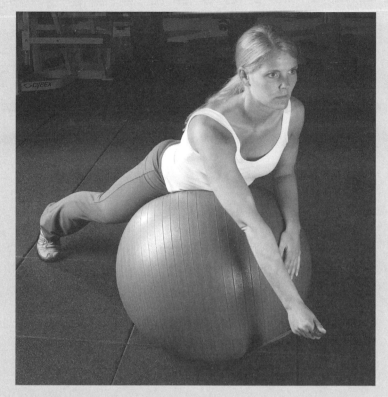

Starting position.

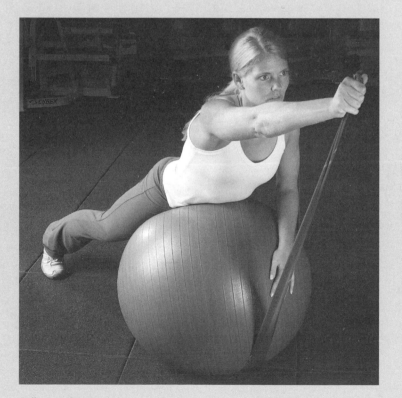

Pull up and extend your arm.

Self-Mobilization with Physioball and Foam Roller

BENEFITS: *Upper-back strength, posture*

Equipment

- Large physioball
- Three-foot-long round foam roller

How do I do this?

1. Lie on your back with your calves on top of the physioball. Your thighs should be in front of the ball and squeezing together, with your hips on the floor.

2. Place the foam roller under you, just beneath your shoulder blades.

3. Place your hands behind your head and curl your trunk slightly forward, pressing your lower back into the floor.

4. Tilt your head all the way back to the floor, allowing your lower back to rise. You'll feel the foam roller pressing into the middle of your back.

5. Perform seven to ten repetitions.

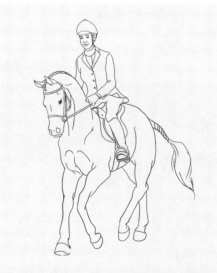

This important mobilizing exercise helps to create extension in the upper regions of the spine and assists in keeping your back straight while mounted.

HINTS

- Concentrate on curling your trunk and flattening your lower back into the floor.
- Keep your head still and in place.

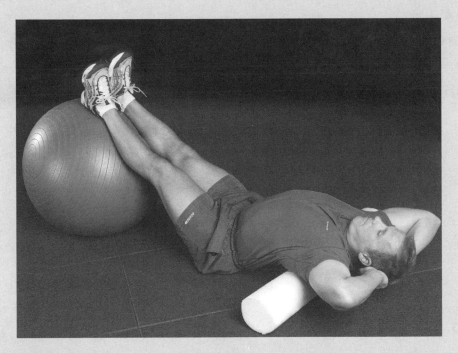

Starting position.

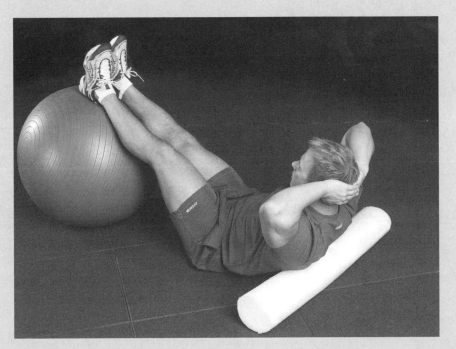

Trunk curl.

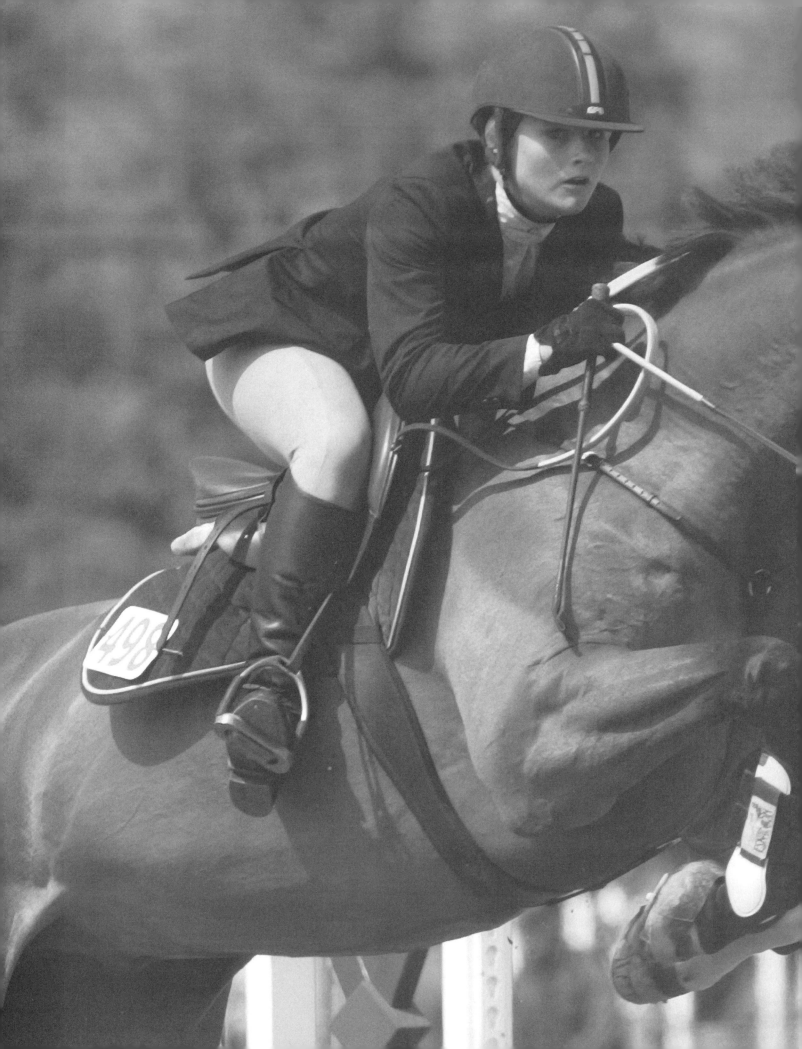

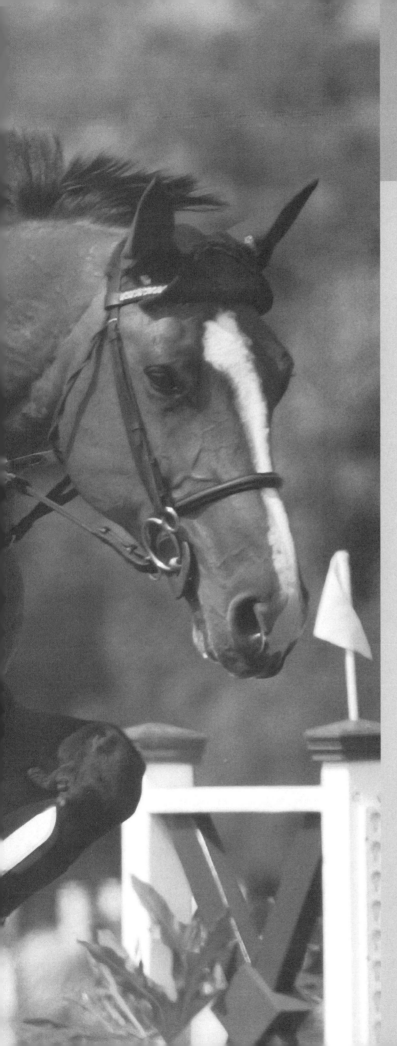

Chapter 6

UPPER BODY

Your upper body is a bastion of strength and stability; shoulder strength improves upper-body control and posture. A stable upper body is necessary for developing clear communication with your horse through soft and steady hands.

Poor upper-body control can cost you rails in a jumper class, cause an injury on a fresh or green horse, or prevent that all-important lead change when you really need it. A polo player swings a mallet to hit a small ball; a hunt servant cracks a whip to stop rioting hounds. Your muscles need to be strong to maintain your posture and balance, as well as control of your horse, while performing mounted tasks.

Upper-body strength is also helpful off the horse. Longeing, driving, grooming, cleaning stalls, and building courses are all activities that are more easily completed with good upper-body strength.

Bench Press

BENEFIT: *Shoulder strength*

Equipment

- Weight bar and bench or bench press
- Small blocks (optional)

How do I do this?

1. Lie on your back on the bench and position your feet comfortably on the floor. Your thighs should be parallel to the floor, or slightly above parallel. If you are short and your thighs angle toward the floor, place small blocks under your feet to achieve the correct position.

2. Hold the bar at approximately shoulder width and lower it toward your chest. Your elbows should be positioned comfortably, about 12 inches from your body.

3. Push the bar straight up until your arms straighten above you.

4. Pause for 1 second, then carefully return the bar to your chest.

5. Perform seven to ten repetitions.

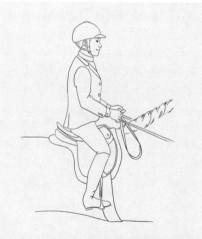

The Bench Press is a standard exercise for developing strength around your shoulders. Balanced tension around the shoulder joint leads to improved posture and function and a better riding position.

HINTS

- Be sure to pull your shoulders back down to the bench prior to returning to the starting position.
- Keep the bar steady, resisting gravity, when lowering it toward your chest.
- When pushing up, pick a spot above you and move deliberately toward that target.

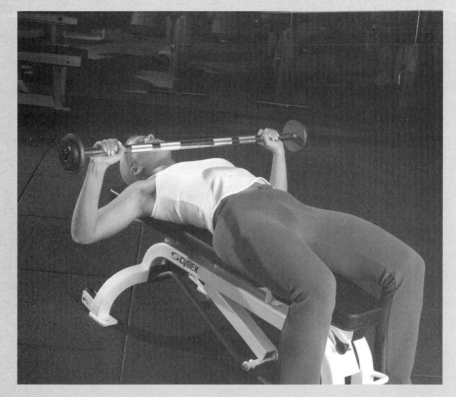

Weight bar at shoulder width.

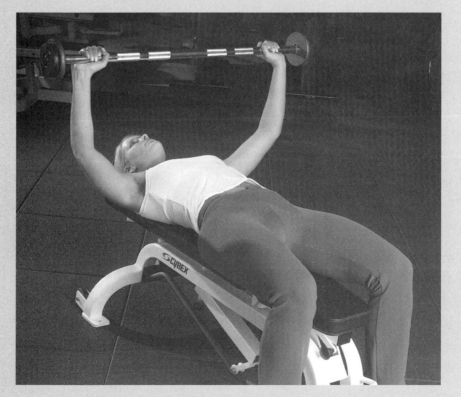

Push bar straight up.

Close-Grip Bench Press

BENEFIT: *Function in the small muscle groups of the shoulder*

Equipment

- Bench
- Weight bar or dumbbells
- Small blocks (optional)

How do I do this?

1. Lie on your back on a bench and position your feet comfortably on the floor. Your thighs should be parallel to the floor, or slightly above parallel. If your thighs angle toward the floor, place small blocks under your feet to achieve the correct position.

2. With your arms by your sides, grab the bar so your wrists are positioned directly above your elbows.

3. Push the bar straight up until your arms are straight above you.

4. Pause for 1 second, then carefully return the bar to your chest.

5. Perform seven to ten repetitions.

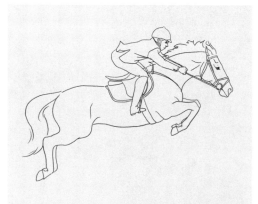

The Close-Grip Bench Press improves your shoulder function, emphasizing some of the smaller muscle groups around the shoulder joint. It also approximates your arm position during riding and will contribute to improved control when mounted.

HINTS

- Be sure to pull your shoulders back down to the bench prior to returning to the starting position.
- Focus on moving from the shoulders, with the elbow motion secondary.
- Keep the bar steady, resisting gravity, when lowering it toward your chest.
- When pushing up, pick a spot above you and move deliberately toward that target.

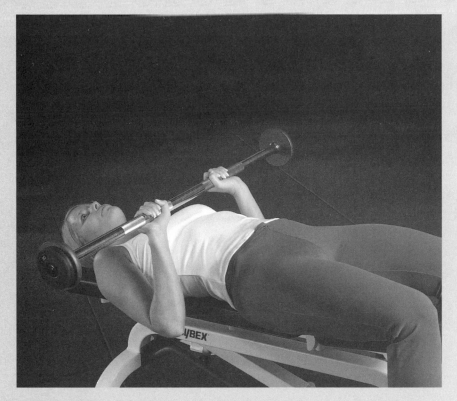

Starting position with close grip.

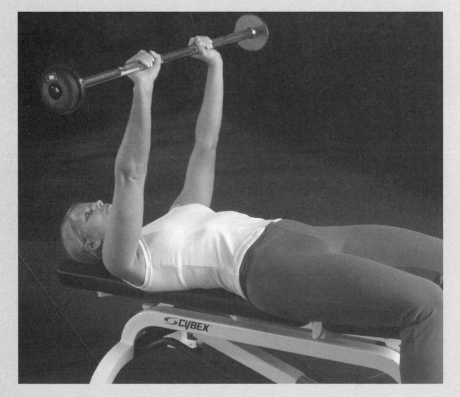

Push bar straight up.

Close-Grip Bench Press, Feet Up

BENEFITS: *Function of the small muscle groups in the shoulder*

Equipment

- Bench
- Weight bar or dumbbells

How do I do this?

1. Lie on your back on a bench.

2. Pull up your legs so your thighs are pointing straight up, your knees are bent, and your feet are pointing toward the ceiling.

3. With your arms by your sides, grab the bar so your wrists are positioned directly above your elbows.

4. Push the bar straight up until your arms are straight above you.

5. Pause for 1 second, then carefully return the bar to your chest.

6. Perform seven to ten repetitions.

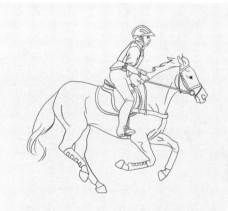

The Close-Grip Bench Press improves your shoulder function, emphasizing some of the smaller muscle groups around the shoulder joint. Elevating the feet creates a slightly less stable position, resulting in improved body control, which will translate to better riding.

HINTS

- Be sure to pull down your shoulders prior to returning to starting position.
- Focus on moving from the shoulders, with the elbow motion secondary.
- Keep the bar steady, resisting gravity, when lowering it toward your chest.
- When pushing up, pick a spot above you and move deliberately toward that target.
- Pay close attention to weight shifts from side to side, and try to prevent your torso from moving.

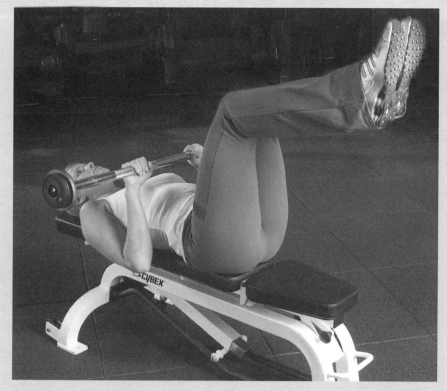

Starting position with feet elevated.

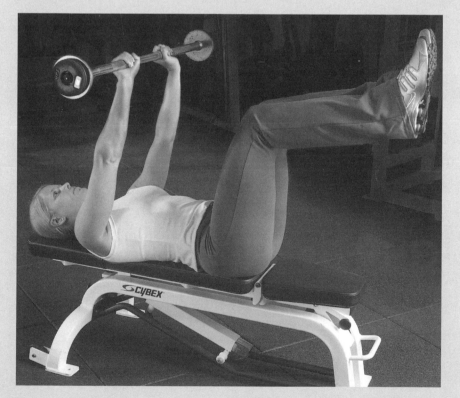

Push bar straight up.

Medicine Ball Push-Up

BENEFITS: *Upper-body strength, posture*

Equipment

- Medicine ball, 8 to 10 inches in diameter
- Mat

How do I do this?

1. Assume a standard push-up position and place your hands on the ball so that they are slightly off-set from center. The middle of your sternum should be directly over the ball, with your elbows a short distance from your sides.

2. Push down into the ball to move your body upward. Continue until your arms are straight. Your body should maintain a straight line. Do not arch your back or let your hips sag.

3. Pause for 1 second, then slowly lower yourself to the starting position.

4. Perform seven to ten repetitions.

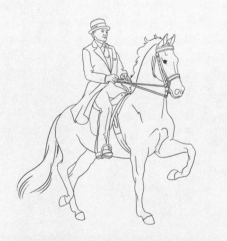

The Medicine Ball Push-up combines upper-body strengthening with postural control. The stabilizing effects of this exercise result in better control and increased confidence when mounted.

HINTS

- Imagine creating a plank with your body to establish postural control.
- Focus on pushing equally with both arms to avoid lateral motion in the ball.
- If the standard exercise is too difficult, try doing a modified push-up on your knees.

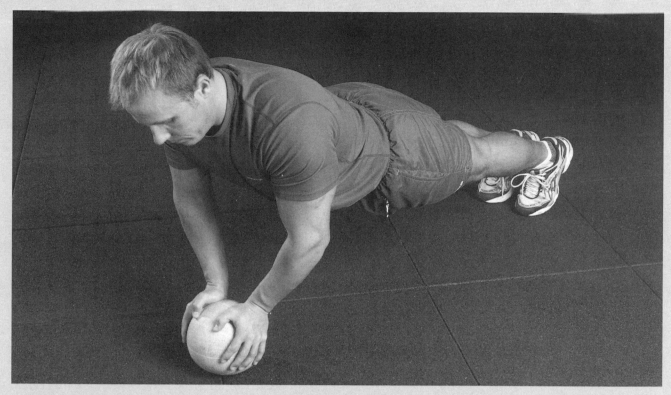

Push down on the ball to move your body upward.

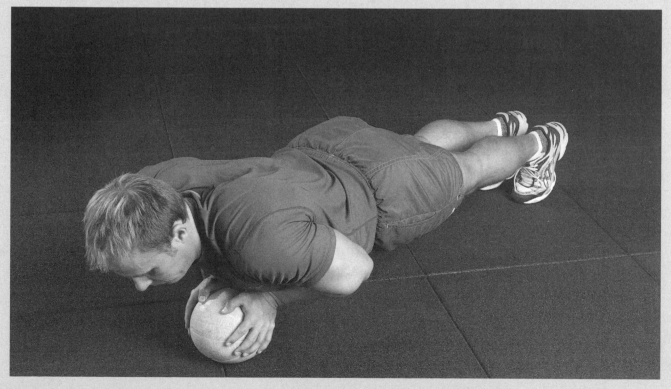

Slowly return to starting position.

Walkover Push-Up

BENEFITS: *Shoulder function, posture*

Equipment

- Mat

How do I do this?

1. Assume a standard push-up position with your body elevated and your arms extended.

2. Lift your left arm and cross it over your right arm, placing your left hand on the floor to the outside of your right hand.

3. As your left hand makes contact with the floor, lower yourself toward the floor, placing equal weight on both hands.

4. Push hard into the floor to elevate your body. As your body begins to move away from the floor, swing your right arm back to the right. This will uncross your arms and bring you back to starting position.

5. Perform seven to ten repetitions with the right arm crossed, then repeat with the left.

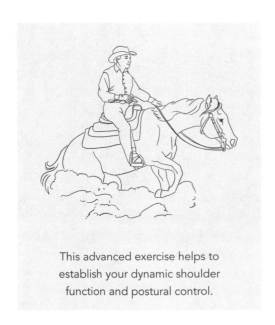

This advanced exercise helps to establish your dynamic shoulder function and postural control.

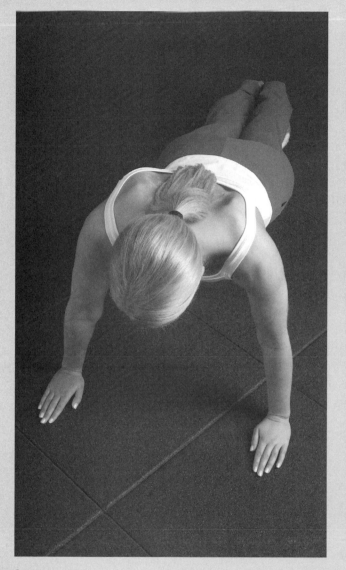

Starting position.

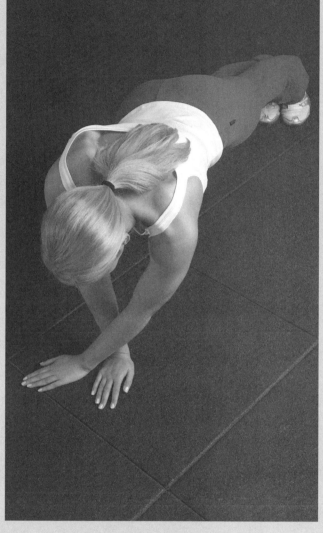

Cross over and lower.

HINTS

- Think about moving your body across the floor as well as up and down.
- Imagine creating a plank with your body to establish postural control.
- Keep your head in a neutral position, facing the floor.
- If the standard exercise is too difficult, try doing a modified push-up on your knees.

Reverse-Grip Pull-Down

BENEFITS: *Shoulders, posture*

Equipment

- Pull-down device
- Elastic tubing or band and stationary stool

Setup

- Secure the tubing to a stable point overhead so that either end of the tubing hangs down.
- Position your stool underneath and grasp each end of the tubing as you would the pull-down bar.

How do I do this?

1. Sit facing the pull-down device. Maintain a tall trunk position.

2. With the palms of your hands facing you, reach up and grab the pull-down bar. Your shoulders, elbows, and wrists should create a vertical line.

3. Focusing on shoulder movement, pull the bar straight down until it is lowered just past your chin.

4. Pause for 1 second, then carefully allow the bar to return to the starting position.

5. Perform seven to ten repetitions.

The Reverse-Grip Pull-Down is an important functional exercise for the shoulders, helping you improve rein control and posture. It also complements the push-up exercises, helping to establish balanced tension around the shoulders.

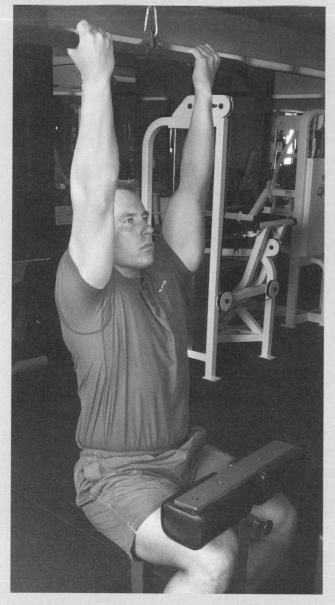

Grab the bar.

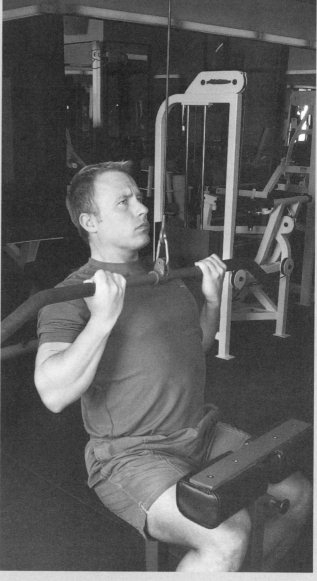

Pull down to below chin.

HINTS

- Keep your hips solidly on the seat.
- Be sure to pull your shoulders down before pulling the bar down.
- Keep your back straight and tall at all times, as if mounted.

Dips

BENEFIT: *Upper-body strength*

Equipment

- Parallel dip bars

How do I do this?

1. Step into the device.

2. Keeping your posture erect, place your hands on the bars so your thumbs are directly over the top pointing forward.

3. Rotate your hands approximately 1 inch from the middle, so your thumbs move to the inside of the center line of the bars.

4. Straighten your arms and lift your feet from the floor so that your body weight is supported entirely by your arms.

5. Slowly lower yourself straight down as far as is comfortable.

6. Push down hard into the bars to return your body to the starting position.

7. Perform seven to ten repetitions.

Dips help establish your dynamic upper-body strength, creating an effective balance between your muscles to the front and the rear of the shoulder.

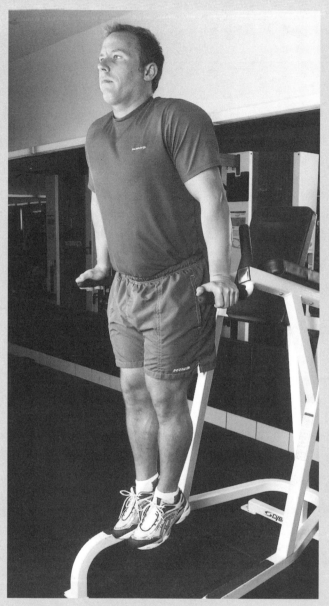

Straight arms support body weight (step 4).

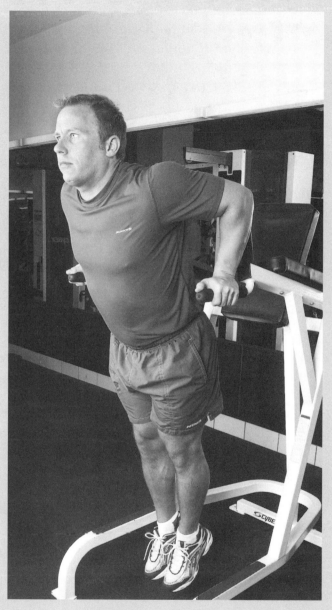

Lower straight down (step 5).

HINTS

- Keep your trunk quiet and your body erect, preventing any forward or backward swaying.
- You can modify this exercise by using a weight-assisted device or by positioning a small stool beneath you on which you can rest your legs, thus providing some additional support.

Straight-Arm Pull-Down

BENEFIT: *Posterior shoulder muscles*

Equipment

- High pulley or elastic tubing, attached at a height of approximately 7 feet

How do I do this?

1. Stand facing the high pulley, approximately 2 feet from the device. If using tubing, stand 2 feet from its point of attachment. Your legs should be shoulder-length apart with your knees slightly bent.

2. Lean forward slightly and grab the pulley handle or tubing with one hand, keeping your arm outstretched. Your arm and shoulder should create a straight line pointing at the pulley or tube attachment.

3. With your body in balance and your arm straight, pull the handle or tubing down and behind you in one long, sweeping arc.

4. Pull as far back as you can without discomfort in your shoulder.

5. Pause for 1 second, then carefully return to the starting position.

6. Perform seven to ten repetitions, then repeat with the other arm.

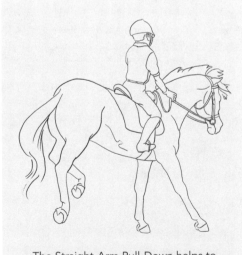

The Straight-Arm Pull-Down helps to develop your posterior shoulder muscles, which are important for improving your posture and increasing your body control.

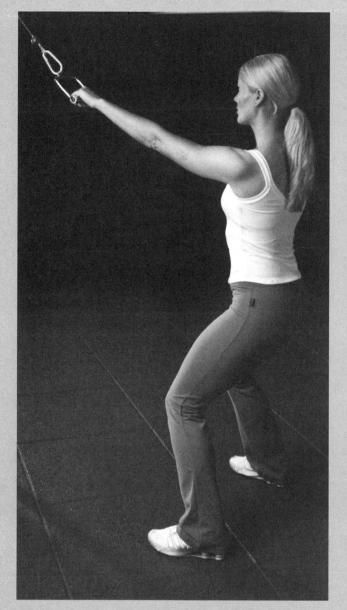

Starting position.

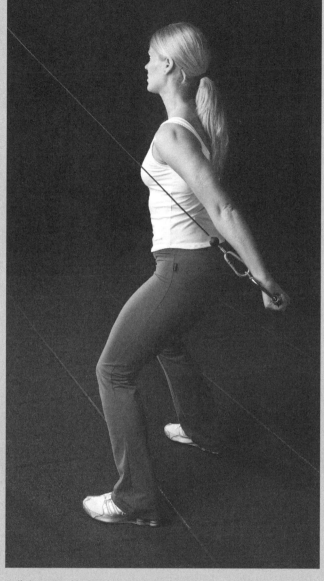

Pull down and behind.

HINT

- Keep your body still with your back straight and your head in a neutral position, aligned with your spine.

Standing Row, Half-Seat Position

BENEFIT: Posture

Equipment

- Adjustable pulley system with a twin rope handle, set at shoulder height, or elastic tubing, anchored at shoulder height in the middle so there are two strands

How do I do this?

1. Stand facing the pulley or tubing anchor point. Your feet should be slightly wider than shoulder width.

2. Grasp the pulley rope handles or the tubing ends and step away from the pulley or anchor point so the cable or tubing is taut. Stretch out your arms in front of you.

4. Assume a half-seat position; the cable or tubing should remain taut. If it slackens, move farther away from the anchor point. Your arms should remain straight in front of you.

5. Keeping your back straight and your head up, pull the handles toward you, leading with your elbows, so your hands come in by your sides.

6. Pause for 1 second, then slowly return the handle to the starting position, remaining in your half-seat.

7. Perform seven to ten repetitions.

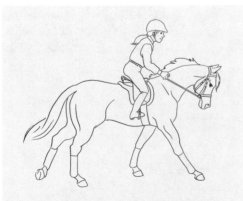

The Standing Row in a half-seat is an excellent exercise for establishing postural control and a good riding position. It is particularly useful in improving your ability to resist forces that pull you forward onto your horse.

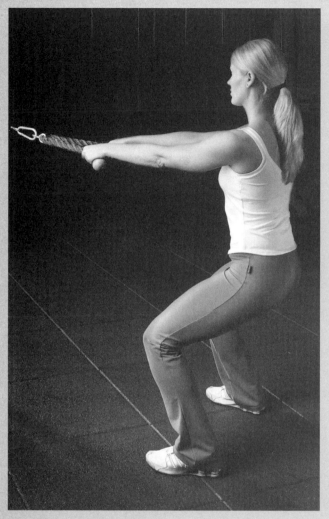

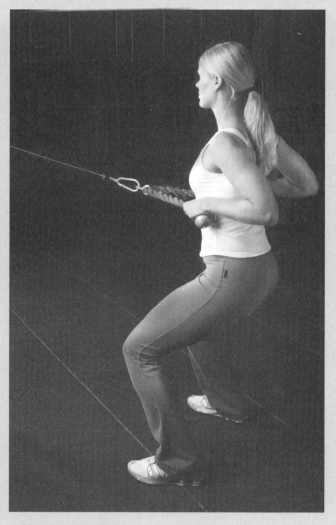

Starting in a half-seat position.

Pull handles toward you.

HINTS

- Focus on remaining balanced on your feet, with your weight centered.
- Be sure to pull back your shoulders to the starting position before moving your arms.

Seated Row, Prone Grip

BENEFIT: *Shoulder strength*

Equipment

- Bench or stool
- Adjustable pulley system, set level with your shoulder, or elastic tubing, anchored in the middle and set level with your shoulder

CHALLENGE

Using a physioball rather than the bench or stool increases the difficulty of this exercise.

How do I do this?

1. Sit on a bench or stool and face the pulley or tubing anchor point. Your feet should be slightly wider than shoulder width.

2. Grasp the pulley rope handles or the tubing ends and sit upright so the cable or tubing is taut. Your arms should be stretched out in front of you.

3. Keeping your back straight and your head up, pull the handles toward you, leading with your elbows, so that your hands come in by your sides.

4. Pause for 1 second, then slowly return the handle to the starting position.

5. Perform seven to ten repetitions.

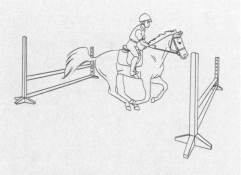

The Seated Row develops posterior shoulder strength, improving your control over the reins. Because the exercise is done in a seated position, greater emphasis is placed on trunk position and postural control, translating to better balance in the saddle.

HINTS

- Focus on remaining balanced and keeping an erect posture.
- Keep your pelvis and spine straight, with your head up.
- Your shoulders may press forward as you reach the starting position. Be sure to pull back your shoulders before moving your arms.

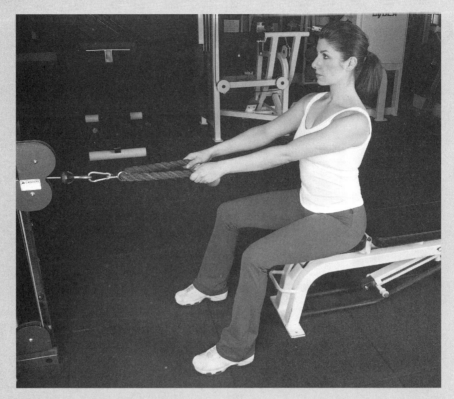

Starting position — arms extended.

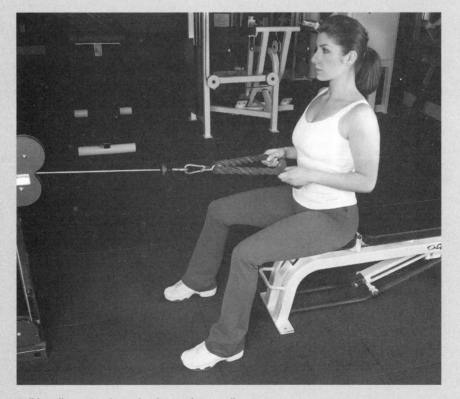

Pull handles toward you, leading with your elbows.

Bent-Over Row

BENEFIT: *Posterior shoulder muscles*

Equipment

- Chair, bench, or physioball
- Dumbbell

CHALLENGE

Using the physioball increases the difficulty of this exercise.

How do I do this?

1. Bend forward from the hips until your upper body is almost parallel to the floor with one arm and leg positioned on the chair, bench, or physioball for support.

2. Grasp a dumbbell in your free hand.

3. Keeping your back flat and your head in a neutral position, let your weighted hand hang straight down toward the floor. Your shoulder may press slightly forward, but be sure your trunk remains level.

4. Pull back your shoulder, then continue pulling the weight straight up, leading with your elbow, positioned close to your side, until the weight is by your side.

5. Pause for 1 second, then slowly lower the weight to the starting position.

6. Perform seven to ten repetitions; repeat on the other side.

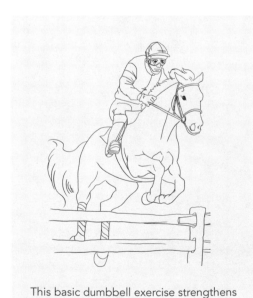

This basic dumbbell exercise strengthens the posterior shoulder muscles, improving control with the reins.

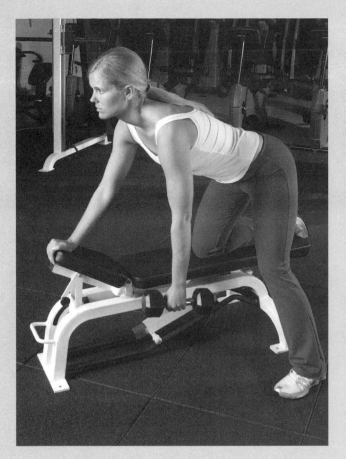

Starting position.

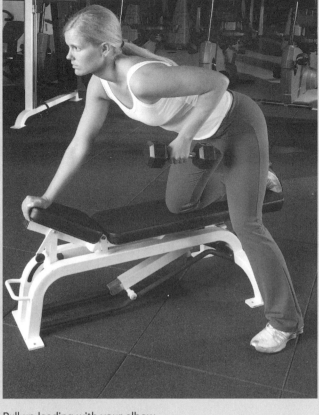

Pull up leading with your elbow.

HINTS

- Keep your trunk still and focus on movement at the shoulder.
- Keep your elbow close to your side.
- Be sure your head is straight; tilting it puts unnecessary strain on the neck.

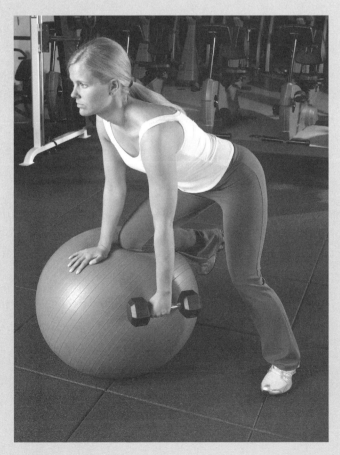

Challenge setup.

Bent-Over Transverse Row

BENEFIT: *Shoulder strength*

Equipment

- Dumbbell
- Physioball, chair, or bench

CHALLENGE

Using the physioball increases the difficulty of this exercise.

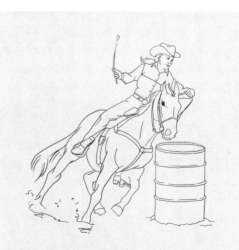

This exercise strengthens your posterior shoulder, shifting the focus of the movement to your smaller shoulder muscles. This is essential for muscular balance around the shoulder joint and overall shoulder function.

How do I do this?

1. With your feet at shoulder width, bend forward from the hips until your body is almost parallel to the floor.

2. Grasp a dumbbell in one hand and use the other arm to support your body weight on the physioball, chair, or bench.

3. Keeping your back flat, spine straight, and head in a neutral position, let your weighted hand hang straight down toward the floor.

4. Pull back your shoulder, then pull the weight straight up, with your elbow pointed away from your side, until the weight is by your side. Your elbow is pointing away from you.

5. Pause for 1 second, then slowly lower the weight to the starting position.

6. Perform seven to ten repetitions; repeat on the other side.

HINTS

- Keep your trunk still and focus on movement at the shoulder.
- Be sure to keep your head in a neutral position; tilting puts unnecessary strain on the neck.
- Your forearm should point straight to the ground throughout the exercise.

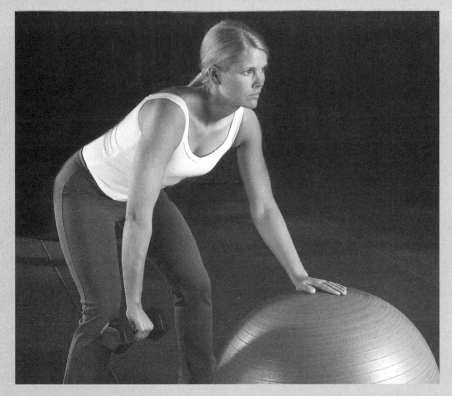

Starting position.

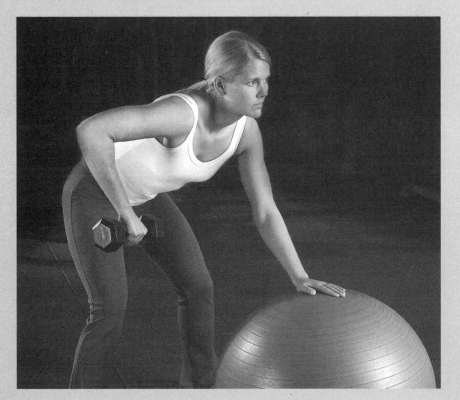

Pull up weight with your shoulder back and elbow pointed out.

Incline Dumbbell Row

BENEFITS: *Shoulders, posture*

Equipment

- Dumbbells
- Bench or physioball

How do I do this?

1. Position your body so that it is tilted approximately 45 degrees toward the floor on an incline bench or physioball.

2. Grasp a dumbbell in each hand and use the bench or physioball to support your weight evenly.

3. Keeping your back flat and your head in a neutral position, let your weighted hands hang straight down toward the floor.

4. Your shoulders may press slightly forward, but be sure to keep your torso flat and your spine straight.

5. Pull back your shoulders, then continue pulling the weights straight up, leading with your elbows, until the weights are by your sides. Your elbows should point away from you.

6. Pause for 1 second, then slowly lower your arms to the starting position.

7. Perform seven to ten repetitions.

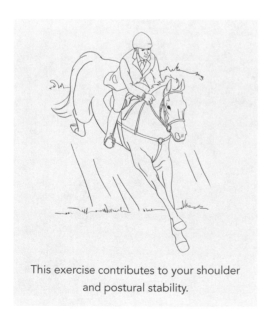

This exercise contributes to your shoulder and postural stability.

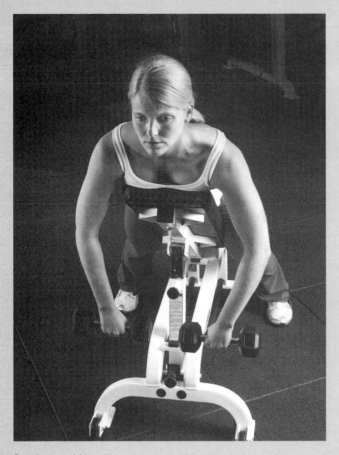

Starting position.

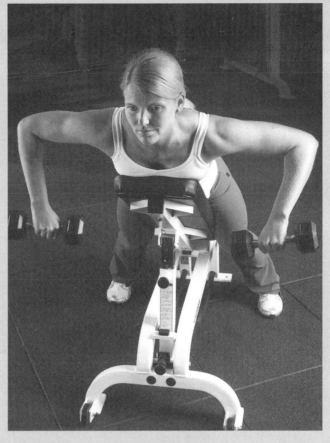

Pull up weights, your elbows pointed out.

HINTS

- Keep your trunk still and focus on movement at the shoulder.
- Be sure to keep your head in a neutral position; tilting puts unnecessary strain on your neck.
- Your forearm should point straight to the ground throughout the exercise.
- The weight should move directly up and down through space, not perpendicular to the angle of your spine.

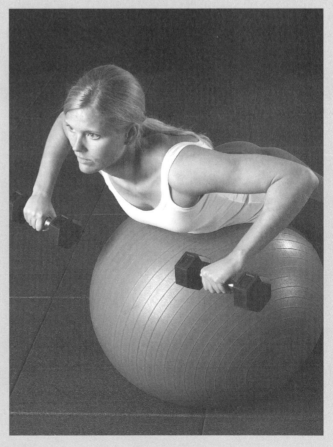

Challenge.

Upright Row

BENEFITS: *Posture, stability*

Equipment

- Dumbbells

How do I do this?

1. Stand tall with your feet at shoulder width.

2. Take a dumbbell in each hand and position them together in front of you, at your waist.

3. Shift your body weight to one foot, bending the other leg at the knee.

4. Keeping your torso still, pull the weights directly up toward your chin, leading with your elbows. Your elbows should be higher than your shoulders and pointing out to the sides.

5. Pause for 1 second, then slowly lower the weights to starting position.

6. Perform seven to ten repetitions.

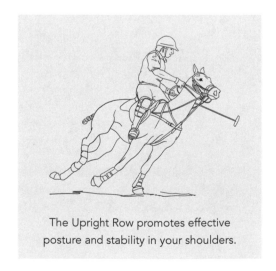

The Upright Row promotes effective posture and stability in your shoulders.

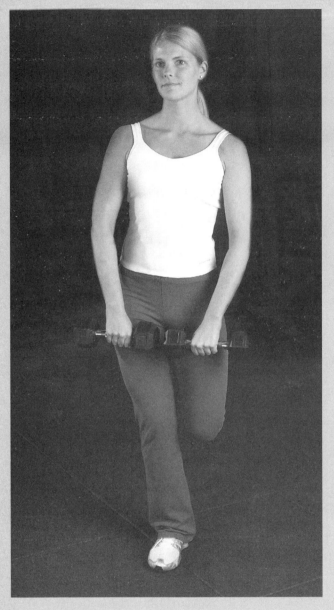

Starting position.

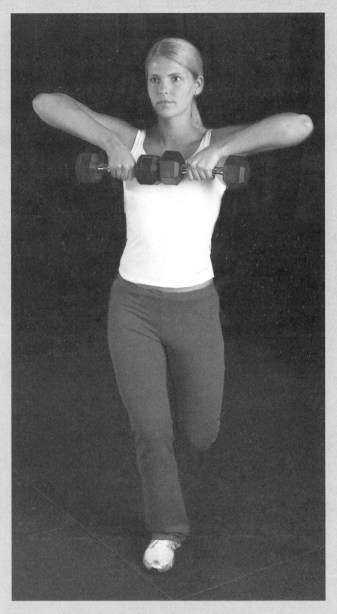

Raise weights to chin, leading with your elbows.

HINT

- Keep the knee of your supporting leg slightly bent to establish a balanced posture.

GLOSSARY

Abductor/adductor. Muscles that control the inward (adduction) and outward (abduction) movements of the hips and shoulders. They are particularly important stabilizers of the hip, an area where flexibility, strength, and control are critical. Abductors move the leg away from the body and adductors move the leg toward the body. When working together, these two muscle groups keep the leg in a fixed position, providing stability to the rider.

Absorbing energy. The ability to become part of the horse's movement. The hips, lower back, and pelvis must be both strong and flexible to accomplish this. Compare to *Transmitting energy.*

Aerobic (cardiovascular). The fitness of the heart and lungs. This is important for all riders, regardless of skill level, and especially important when training, competing, or working at speed or over fences.

Asymmetry/asymmetric. Unequal or different movement on the two sides of the body; using only one side of the body to execute riding aids. Compare to *Symmetry/symmetric.*

Center of gravity (COG). The critical focal point for the body's balance. COG depends on a person's size and shape. When mounted, the rider's center of gravity should match the horse's. As the gait or speed changes, the horse's COG changes; thus; so does the rider's upper-body position. A properly trained dressage horse has a very upright COG at all gaits; a racehorse has a more forward COG.

Closed skill. A skill that is highly predictable. The conditions requiring the skill do not change; therefore, the training required involves perfecting a predictable task. Compare to *Open skill.*

Core stability. The rider's ability to maintain balance and position while mounted, regardless of the horse's actions.

Countercanter (canter on the counter-lead). A training exercise in which the horse holds the outside leading leg and corresponding bend in the body while executing a smooth, not sharp, turn in the opposite direction. The countercanter is an excellent example of a rider's need for asymmetric multitasking.

Ducking. An exaggerated and quick movement of the rider's torso forward or down on the horse's neck as the horse jumps. Being strong and fit and having a secure leg helps prevent this upper-body problem.

Dynamic posture. A characteristic of good riding posture. Because the rider and horse are constantly in motion, the rider's posture will change frequently. The ability to be dynamic in the saddle is closely related to physical fitness.

FEI (Fédération Equestre Internationale). The international governing body for equestrian sports.

Flying change. A lead maneuver in which the horse canters or gallops and, during the suspension phase of a stride, switches from one leading leg to the other. See also *Leads.*

Focus. A calm and directed concentration on the task at hand. Focus encourages precision and accuracy in communicating with the horse while riding. Practicing multitasking exercises helps develop focus.

Full seat. A riding position in which the weight of the upper body is carried in the saddle through a supple yet straight, nearly vertical back. The ultimate use of the full seat is in dressage.

Functional flexibility. The flexibility required to perform the functions of a task.

Galloping position (*Half-seat* or *Two-point position*). A riding position in which the rider holds his or her seat above the saddle, with all of the body's weight centered over the legs. The half-seat is used in training to secure and strengthen the leg position, as well as in competition when the horse requires total freedom from weight on his back.

Getting ahead. When the rider shifts his or her balance forward of the horse's center of gravity. This often occurs prior to the horse pushing off the ground at a jump.

Half-seat. See *Galloping position.*

Leads. A horse is on the correct lead when his inside shoulder is slightly further forward than his outside shoulder. A good rider can tell this by the way her hips move. If the horse is on the correct lead the rider's outside hip will turn slightly to the inside.

Left behind. Falling behind the motion or balance of the horse. Compare to *Getting ahead.*

Light seat. The basic, most frequently used position for jumping. The rider's weight is distributed primarily into the legs, through nonrigid hips, knees, and ankles down to the heel, while the rider's seat maintains light forward contact with the saddle.

Lumbar region. The lower spine, which acts as a shock absorber, especially at the sitting trot and canter.

Multitasking. Acting on and processing information simultaneously. When riding, the legs, arms, shoulders, back, seat, and head are usually performing different actions.

Open skill. A skill that is highly unpredictable and rapidly changing. Compare to *Closed skill.*

Pelvic absorption. The ability of the pelvic area (hips, pelvis, and lumbar region) to absorb shock, such as at the trot or canter.

Plantar stabilizers. The hips, knees, and ankles; often compared to shock absorbers.

Rhythm. The tempo of a horse's gait. Maintaining rhythm indicates a horse that is not changing pace and is proceeding forward with a regular and consistent tempo.

The rider has a direct influence on the horse's ability to achieve, maintain, and regain a good rhythm.

Symmetry/symmetric. Even and square posture; when both sides of the body are performing a balanced action. For example: Walking is a symmetrical exercise, even though the actions of your arms and legs are diametric. Compare to *Asymmetry/ asymmetric.*

Squat position. A standing posture in which the lower back is arched, the knees are bent, and the feet are flat on the ground.

Transmitting energy. How the rider uses the energy generated by the horse. Compare to *Absorbing energy.*

Two-point position. See *Galloping position.*

Visualizing. A valuable sports psychology technique in which the rider completes a mental run-through of every aspect of an exercise prior to actually executing it. This technique can be extremely helpful in preparing for competition.

RESOURCES

Our Web site

For more information on equestrian fitness and author events please visit our Web site **www.ridinghighfitness.com**. All of the fitness products used in this program can be purchased at ridinghighfitness.com. We offer a variety of products for all fitness levels and activities, and provide professional instruction on the set-up and proper use of products. Our team of leading fitness experts is available online five days a week to provide one-on-one support and customer service to assist you in your fitness endeavors. Additional copies of the pull-out cards included in this book are also available online.

Fitness Books

This is a selection of the many books on horse and rider fitness, as well as of books on riding and showing in general. Beginning your library with these will give you a head start in your equestrian education.

Most of these can be ordered from your local bookstore or one of the online retailers. Titles not available in the United States may be found on one of the British booksellers' Web sites.

In most countries, there are also excellent weekly and monthly periodicals offering ongoing articles on training.

Barron's Atlas of Anatomy. New York: Barron's Educational Series, Inc. 1995.
This small book has excellent color illustrations of human anatomy and is useful in understanding how your body performs while exercising.

Benedik, Linda, and Veronica Wirth. *Yoga for Equestrians.* North Pomfret, VT: Trafalgar Square, 2000.
All disciplines are incorporated into this program of Yoga for equestrians, which is aimed at helping you build a stronger mind–body connection for improved performance.

Bromily, Mary. *Fit to Ride.* Oxford, UK and Malden, MA: Blackwell Science, 2000.
A wonderful book that combines rider fitness with horse fitness.

Holderness-Roddam, Jane. *Fitness for Horse and Rider: Gain More from Your Riding by Improving Your Horse's Fitness and Condition — and Your Own.* Devon, UK: David & Charles, 1997.
Another book from an experienced competitor and writer that combines the fitness of horse and rider. Out of print in the United States, but still available from J. A. Allen in England.

Holmes, Tom. *The New Total Rider: Health and Fitness for Equestrians.* Boonesboro, MD: Half Halt Press, 2001.

A very good book on equestrian fitness, with exercises and nutritional information.

Midkiff, Mary. *Fitness, Performance, and the Female Equestrian.* Hoboken, NJ: Howell Book House, 1996.

An interesting discourse that focuses on women's unique physical challenges, from the way the pelvis is constructed to the problems inherent in aging and childbirth and how they affect female riders. Also includes specific exercises, a discussion of injury prevention around the barn, and a good section on nutrition.

Pilliner, Sarah, and Zoe Davies. *Getting Horses Fit: A Guide to Improved Performance*, third edition. Oxford, UK, and Malden, MA: Blackwell Science, 2000.

Sometimes in our eagerness to get fit, we forget that our horses also need to be fit and ready for competition. This is a thorough and scientific study of equine fitness and its relationship to health problems, and how to manage it all.

Steiner, Betsy, and Jennifer O. Bryant. *Gymnastic Dressage Training Using Mind, Body, and Spirit.* Buckingham, UK: Kenilworth Press, 2003.

An extraordinarily beautiful book, and certainly a must-read for anyone interested in dressage. The authors combine the mind, body, and spirit of horses and riders with a selection of physical and mental exercises both mounted and dismounted.

von Dietze, Susanne. *Balance in Movement: The Seat of the Rider.* North Pomfret, VT: Trafalgar Square, 1999.

Originally published in German, this book is an excellent study of what happens where in our bodies when we ride.

Books on Riding

Allen, Linda L., and Dianna Dennis. *101 Jumping Exercises for Horses and Riders.* North Adams, MA: Storey Publishing, 2003.

A must-read for anyone interested in English riding, even those who do not jump but especially for those who do.

Bayley, Lesley, and Caroline Davis. *The Less-Than-Perfect Rider: Overcoming Common Riding Problems.* Hoboken, NJ: Howell Book House, 1994.

The demands and frustrations of riding are discussed in this sensible approach to conquering real or imagined physical and emotional inadequacies. A well-developed and useful treatise.

Campion, Lynn. *Training and Showing the Cutting Horse.* Guilford, CT: The Lyons Press, 2000.

Riding a cutting horse requires all the strength, balance, and coordination a rider can muster. This book is great for anyone, whether a beginner or more experienced, who wants to try cutting.

Delmar, Diana. *Taking Up Riding as an Adult.* North Adams, MA: Storey Publishing, 1998.

This is especially useful for the adult beginner.

d'Endrody, Lt. Col. A. L. *Give Your Horse a Chance.* London: J. A. Allen, 1989 (rev. 1999).

A classic book, with excellent sections on training and conditioning the jumper and event horse.

deNemethy, Bertlan. *The deNemethy Method.* New York: Doubleday, 1988 (rev. 1999).

As USET Show Jumping coach from 1952 to 1984, deNemethy molded the American jumping style and took it to its peak. A must for every jumping fan.

Dunning, Al. *Reining.* Guilford, CT: The Lyons Press, 2002.

Considered the bible of Western reining.

Harris, Susan E. *The United States Pony Club Manuals of Horsemanship.* Hoboken, NJ: Howell Book House, 1994–1996.

These thorough manuals consist of *The United States Pony Club Manual of Horsemanship — Basics for Beginners, D Level* (1994), *The United States Pony Club Manual of Horsemanship — Intermediate Horsemanship, C Level* (1995), and *The United States Pony Club Manual of Horsemanship — B, HA, A Levels* (1996).

Hill, Cherry. *Becoming an Effective Rider: Develop Your Mind and Body for Balance and Unity.* North Adams, MA: Storey Publishing, 1991.

How to achieve maximum benefit from lessons, improve communication with the horse, use riding-safety principles, and overcome some common rider hurdles. Especially useful for the beginner or returning rider.

Jackson, Noel. *Effective Horsemanship.* New York: Arco Publishing, 1967.

An older (and out-of-print) book that has a lot of excellent information about jumping and about training the jumping horse.

Kursinski, Anne. *Anne Kursinski's Riding and Jumping Clinic.* New York: Doubleday and Co., 1995.

Riding champion Kursinski trained under the late Jimmy Williams, then moved to George Morris. She is classic in her approach and explains well.

Littauer, Vladimer S. *The Forward Seat.* Lanham, MD: Derrydale Press, 1937.

One of the early proponents of the forward seat here in America. This is one of the first books on the subject.

Morris, George. *Hunter Seat Equitation.* New York: Doubleday and Co., 1979.

An absolute must-have from the god of the hunter-jumper world.

O'Connell, Alice L. *The Blue Mare in the Olympic Trials.* Boston: G. P. Putnam and Sons, 1956.
Pamela and the Blue Mare. Boston: G. P. Putnam and Sons, 1952.

These two little novels detail the training of a horse from the ground up. Dressage, gymnastic jumping, and cross-country riding are all covered and very understandable. Does your child/student not really understand gymnastics and the importance of flatwork? These books explain it all and tell a lovely story as well. Vladimer Littauer and Colonel Wofford (Jimmy Wofford's father and an Olympian) were the technical advisers for these novels.

Paalman, Anthony. *Training Showjumpers.* London: J. A. Allen, 1998.

This is one of the most interesting, classic, and comprehensive books ever written on riding and jumping. A must for any serious equestrian library.

Richter, Judy. *Horse and Rider.* New York: Doubleday and Co., 1984.

Richter, a graduate "A" Pony Clubber, is a veteran trainer on the show circuit and has been called one of the best teachers in the business. An English teacher before becoming a full-time professional equestrian instructor, she has written a clear and easy-to-use basic manual.

Shrake, Richard. *Western Horsemanship: The Complete Guide to Riding the Western Horse.* Guilford, CT: The Lyons Press, 2002.

This complete guide to riding Western takes the student from training to showing and teaching and judging.

Steinkraus, William. *Riding and Jumping.* New York: Doubleday and Co., 1969.

A book of riding and philosophy from the 1968 Olympic gold-medal winner. Another important book, along with its sequel, *Reflections on Riding and Jumping* (1991).

Strickland, Charlene. *The Basics of Western Riding.* North Adams, MA: Storey Publishing, 1998.

A good primer for the beginner Western rider, or for someone who is going on that horsey vacation.

Wofford, James. *Training the Three-Day Event Horse and Rider.* New York: Doubleday Equestrian Library, 1995.

Not just for the event horse and rider! Excellent exercises presented in an easy format. Lots of discussion of fitness and flatwork—both essential for any type of riding.

Wright, Gordon. *Learning to Ride, Show and Hunt.* New York: Doubleday, 1966.

A classic in the field. Wright was George Morris's teacher and mentor.

INDEX

Page numbers in **bold** indicate a box.
Page numbers in *italic* indicate an illustration or photograph.

ABOUT THE AUTHORS   ACKNOWLEDGMENTS

Dianna Robin Dennis is a lifelong equestrian, writer, and frequent contributor to equestrian publications, including *Chronicle of the Horse, Equestrian Magazine, Horse Illustrated,* and *Horse People.* She is the coauthor of *101 Jumping Exercises for Horse and Rider.*

John J. McCully is a certified fitness professional and personal trainer. He appears frequently on national and regional television, and speaks at conferences and seminars across the country. His articles have appeared in magazines and newspapers including *Fitness Magazine, Men's Journal,* and *Practical Horseman.* John is cofounder of Riding High Fitness, an equestrian fitness company that tailors fitness programs for individual riders.

Paul M. Juris is a nationally recognized kinesiologist. His movement-based focus on rehabilitation and performance has been adopted by NBA teams including the New York Knicks, Atlanta Hawks, and Dallas Mavericks. As director of the renowned Equinox Fitness Training Institute of the Equinox Fitness Clubs, Dr. Juris established the most successful personal training program in the fitness industry. Dr. Juris is a frequent lecturer at medical, scientific, sports, and fitness conferences. He is an advisory board member of *Fitness Magazine.*

The authors wish to thank Equinox Fitness Clubs for their support and facilities, Cybex International, Inc., Market Street Inc., Life Fitness, and Precore. Thank you to fitness models Lori Matan and Tracy Jetzer.

Many thanks to the photographers, Jeff Shaffer and Dawn Smith, and to illustrator James Dykeman. Thanks also to Gregg Isaacs for his expert advice and enthusiasm for the project. Special thanks to Deborah Burns and the team at Storey Publishing for helping to shape the program into a book.

Thanks especially to Anne Kursinski and Marion Davidson for being such outstanding examples of passion, integrity, and commitment. Finally, we thank our horses for their patience.

In addition, John McCully would like to thank the following:

My good friends Mike Fitch, Mark Myers, Lori Matan, and Marion Davidson. I thank you all for your support over the years. Thank you to my dear friend David Harris, whose wisdom and unconditional friendship pulled me over the bumpy roads, and whose input I always hold valuable. I am eternally grateful.

To my mentor, Dr. Paul Juris, well, what can I say . . . you're the man!

OTHER STOREY TITLES YOU WILL ENJOY

101 Arena Exercises, by Cherry Hill. Cherry Hill presents recognized classic exercises, suitable for both English and Western riders, along with her own original patterns and maneuvers. ISBN 0-88266-316-X.

101 Jumping Exercises for Horse & Rider, by Linda Allen with Dianna R. Dennis. Provides a logical and consistent series of exercises with clear maps and straightforward instructions. ISBN 1-58017-465-5.

The Horse Doctor Is In, by Brent Kelley, DVM. "This is one of the best veterinary books I've seen in years . . . it is a very readable book for pleasure as well as information." — *The American Quarter Horse Journal*. ISBN 1-58017-460-4.

Horse Handling & Grooming, by Cherry Hill. This user-friendly guide offers a wealth of practical advice on mastering dozens of essential skills. ISBN 0-88266-956-7.

Horsekeeping on a Small Acreage, by Cherry Hill. Design safe, functional stable facilities that meet the needs of your horse. Covers all the necessary steps — from selecting acreage and designing layout to constructing barn and storage facilities. ISBN 0-88266-596-0.

Storey's Guide to Raising Horses, by Heather Smith Thomas. Whether you are an experienced horse handler or are planning to buy your first horse, this complete guide to intelligent horsekeeping covers all aspects of keeping a horse fit and healthy. ISBN 1-58017-127-3.

Storey's Guide to Training Horses, by Heather Smith Thomas. Covering everything from basic safety to retraining a horse that has acquired bad habits, this is an essential handbook for all horse owners. ISBN# 1-58017-467-1

These and other Storey books are available wherever books are sold and directly from Storey Publishing, 210 Mass MoCA Way, North Adams, MA 01247, or by calling 1-800-441-5700. Or visit our Web site at www.storey.com.